MEMORY'S
LAST
BREATH

MEMORY'S LAST BREATH

Field Notes on My Dementia

GERDA SAUNDERS

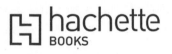
hachette
BOOKS
NEW YORK BOSTON

Hachette Books
Hachette Book Group
1290 Avenue of the Americas
New York, NY 10104
hachettebooks.com
twitter.com/hachettebooks

First edition: June 2017

All images courtesy of the author, except for the following: page 29 Cheryl Saunders; page 79 (top) Cheryl Saunders, adapted from the *Journal of Cosmology*, (5 bottom images) courtesy of Patricia Kinser; page 80 Cheryl Saunders. Images used with permission.

Hachette Books is a division of Hachette Book Group, Inc. The Hachette Books name and logo are trademarks of Hachette Book Group, Inc.

The publisher is not responsible for websites (or their content) that are not owned by the publisher.

The Hachette Speakers Bureau provides a wide range of authors for speaking events. To find out more, go to www.hachettespeakersbureau.com or call (866) 376-6591.

Library of Congress Cataloging-in-Publication Data has been applied for.

ISBNs: 978-0-316-50262-7 (hardcover), 978-0-316-50263-4 (ebook)

Printed in the United States of America

LSC-C

10 9 8 7 6 5 4 3 2 1

For my made-in-America family—now too extended to name—the friends of my heart who are now "blood"

for the Salt Lake City Saunderses: Kanye, Aliya, and Dante, and those people who transport them to visit Ouma and Oupa

and, of course, for Peter: Your name is Rock, where elephants shelter when the heavens frown.

Contents

Author's Note   *ix*

Chapter One: Telling Who I Am before I Forget   1

Chapter Two: Quantum Puff Adders and
      Fractional Memories   14

Chapter Three: The Grammar of the Disappearing Self   47

Chapter Four: This Is Your Brain on the Fritz   74

Chapter Five: Of Madness and Love I   120

Chapter Six: Of Madness and Love II   158

Chapter Seven: Makeovers in Extremis   182

Chapter Eight: The Exit That Dare Not Say Its Name   211

Acknowledgments   257

Notes   259

Author's Note

When I was diagnosed with early-onset dementia just before my sixty-first birthday in 2010, I kept my hurt, anger, fear, and doubts under wraps. I had no choice. I had a job, a husband, children, grandchildren, friends. I had a life. However, there is nothing like a death sentence—in my case, the premature death of my mind—to provoke questions about life. What, actually, is memory, personality, identity? What is a self? Will I still be (have?) a self when my reason is gone? For me, the place to work out such questions has always been in writing. From that place of self-reckoning, then, came this book.

In July 2011—nine months after my diagnosis—when I retired from my position as the associate director of the Gender Studies Program at the University of Utah, my colleagues gave me a beautiful leather-bound journal as a goodbye present. I took to jotting down notes in it about my daily misadventures—pots on the stove boiling dry, washing my hair twice in an hour, forgetting to bake a casserole I had prepared the night before. With a wink at my background in the sciences, I called my journal *Dementia Field Notes*: I would be an anthropologist, assigned to observe one member of a strange tribe, the Dementers. Like a true scientist, I would be objective. No whining, wailing, or gnashing of teeth. Just the facts.

A month or two into my "objective" writing, I also started to write a personal narrative about my dementia. Objectivity be damned. I felt compelled to tell my story from the inside. Months later, the piece turned into an essay. After some tough-love editing by two of my closest friends—Shen Christenson and Kirstin Scott, both writers—I showed the essay to my husband, Peter, my children Marissa and Newton and their spouses, and a few close friends. They urged me to share the essay with others and, to my delight, demanded I write more.

I wrote a second essay, which included summaries of neurological research into various forms of dementia. The idea that my writing might add up to a book slowly started to take shape. Two and a half years after my first *Field Notes* entry, I had completed three essays. I was mentally exhausted. I had little energy left to enjoy my life. My working memory—the ability to hold a small amount of info in my head while using it, such as remembering the street name *and* street number as I wrote down an address while someone said it on the phone—barely functioned. Neuropsychological tests showed a decline in my IQ. I began to question if writing a book was worth these losses. Was this how I wanted to spend my remaining "good years"?

I decided to end my excursion into writing with a bang. Starting in September 2012, I mined my completed essays for passages that would add up to a stand-alone piece for publication. The result was published as "Telling Who I Am before I Forget: My Dementia" in the Winter 2013 issue of the *Georgia Review* (GR) and subsequently reprinted in the large-circulation online magazine *Slate*. That a *Slate* editor would even notice my essay in an academic journal—though it consistently ranks first or near the top of its peers on Pushcart's list of nonfiction journals—had been a matter of great serendipity. But Dan Kois is not just any editor—having started out at *Slate* as culture editor, he made a habit of reading academic journals for reprint possibilities. While Kois cruised the publishers' displays at the 2014 conference of the Association of Writers and Writing Programs, the editor managing GR's booth handed him a copy of the Winter 2013 issue and mentioned my essay, in Dan's words, "as one they were particularly enthusiastic about." (Blessings on the *Georgia Review*'s extraordinary staff!)

To my surprise, the *Slate* essay was reviewed or recommended in publications ranging from an NYU School of Medicine newsletter to *Business Insider* to the *New Yorker*. While this recognition stroked my ego, the comments, questions, and contacts I received from readers expanded my heart, particularly those from people who had dementia in their families. My family had been right in thinking that my writing on dementia could be useful in the world—that perhaps, in exploring my own experience on the page, I could in some way help shed light on the confusion, embarrassments, hurt feelings, and shrinking self-image that many people with dementia experience. Inevitably, my Calvinist upbringing kicked in: It was my *duty* to continue the book. And then, out of the blue, an email arrived one day from the sine qua non Kate Garrick, a literary agent in New York. Under her watchful eye, I wrote more essays. In time, Kate helped me see that they almost added up to an autobiography. But not quite. Large chunks of my life were missing. During the next two years, Kate nursed me through additions and revisions, a process during which I sometimes got so lost in the manuscript that I almost gave up. My reward for going on was that, in the end, my manuscript provided a glimpse into the full arc of my life. In February 2016, Kate sold my manuscript to Hachette Books, where my editor, the thoughtful perfectionist Paul Whitlatch, helped me shape the somewhat flabby manuscript into the book you now hold in your hands.

My book is for this: to add my personal story to the body of science about dementia already accumulated by the lifetime efforts of neuroscientists, neuropsychologists, other medical researchers, and healthcare providers.

My book is for you: whether you or someone you love has dementia, or you're a medical professional, or a person searching for your own self after a huge life change, or someone just plain curious, who—like me—feels that the more you know, the better you're able to love.

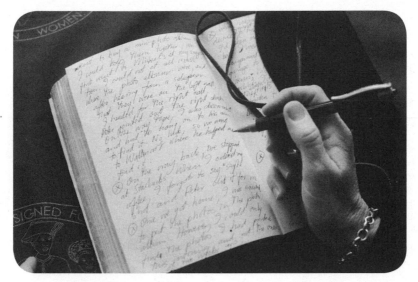

Gerda's Dementia Journal, Vol. I, May 2011–March 2014.

Chapter One

Telling Who I Am before I Forget

ON SEPTEMBER 21, 2010, five days before my sixty-first birthday, I was given a diagnosis of microvascular disease. Following Alzheimer's, microvascular disease is the second leading cause of dementia. I was—as my rather blunt neurologist put it—already "dementing." Insofar as I had thought about dementia before that day, I was unaware that the word had a verb form: *I dement, you dement, he/she/it dements, they dement, we all dement.* Now, six years later, "the cloake sitteth no lesse fit" on my chastened back.

The denial with which I initially met my diagnosis will seem disingenuous in light of the fact that I knew the symptoms of dementia even then—and recognized them in myself. Also, my mother had a form of mental disconnect that made her increasingly out of touch with reality until her death at eighty-two. Given that, why did my doctor's utterance fall so disconsonantly on my ear? It took me a long time to understand how profoundly the diagnosis threatened my sense of identity.

My pursuit of a PhD in English in my forties introduced me to the Enlightenment philosophers. I remember being intrigued by John Locke's and William Whewell's quest for, as Locke puts it, the "originals from whence all our ideas take their beginnings," which took both men back to Adam's expulsion from the Garden of

Eden. Locke describes fallen Adam as lost in a "strange Country" with "all Things new, and unknown about him"; Whewell pictures Adam doing the first work of postlapsarian orientation by giving names "distinct and appropriate to the facts" to newly encountered objects and concepts.

I knew something about this project. Having emigrated in 1984 from South Africa to Salt Lake City with my husband, Peter, and our two children, I had experienced the discombobulation of having to decipher situations that must appear mundane to residents equipped with the requisite cultural vocabulary. What, for example, are you supposed to do when an acquaintance drops by your house with her own beverage in tow? How do two people proceed from acquaintance to friendship without that most crucial foundation of South African hospitality: a fresh pot of tea? Why is letting your kids run naked through the sprinklers in your own backyard or displaying baby pictures of your kids naked regarded by visitors as tantamount to sexual exploitation? What about the forlorn feeling when hosts with whom you have had a marvelous evening say goodbye to you at the door rather than walking you to your car?

By my mid-fifties, I had cracked these and other social codes to a great extent. I knew that having coffee meant heading to the nearest Starbucks. I had built up a scaffolding of friends so dear they had become family. Most of the time I no longer felt like a foreigner. I had developed an American self and was settling into it. But before I had even reached my sixties, I had begun again to feel like an alien of sorts, a stranger even to myself.

I first noted an irksome absentmindedness in my work as the associate director of gender studies at the University of Utah, a position I took at age fifty-two after a foray into the corporate world. Like the troublesome serpent in Genesis, an impairment in my working memory—the ability to maintain and manipulate information "live" in a multistep process, such as remembering to carry the tens when you add numbers—slunk into my intellectual Eden.

My love of teaching was the reason I left my corporate job in 2002 for academics, gladly taking a 25 percent salary cut. After fewer than five years in my dream job, forebodings that not all was well started to cloud my class time: I would lose the thread of a discussion or forget the point toward which I had intended to steer the students' thinking. Often, the name of a novel or author I used to know as well as my children's names would not come to mind. Not infrequently, a student would remind me during the last moments of class that I had failed to distribute notes or an assignment.

I began to prepare scripts for my lessons, but even these did not prevent me from losing my place in my own mnemonic system. Though I had not yet sought a diagnosis, I took our program director into my confidence about my memory difficulties and she graciously supported me in negotiating smaller teaching loads. Soon there was only one class per year. During my last two years of working at the university I was not teaching at all and was instead bogged down in management and meetings, just like in my corporate days.

On the administrative front, too, my fraying memory caused me stress. During the first gathering of a Women's Week committee that I chaired, I had created a detailed agenda to keep me on track: welcome, make introductions, review themes covered in past years, brainstorm ideas for this year, and so forth. At some point between the welcome and the review of previous themes, my mind flipped into confusion. Someone was talking. His voice was distant, and syllables flowed from his mouth without coalescing into meaning. I panicked. I had no idea where we were in the agenda. Desperately scanning my notes, my eye fell on "Introductions." When the speaker paused, I suggested we introduce ourselves. As the words left my mouth, I remembered with horror that we had already gone around the table. My insides cramped at the realization that I had committed the cardinal sin of academia: not thinking accurately on my feet. A colleague from the Women's Resource Center tried to take the edge off my embarrassment by saying that we all had so many things on our plates it was no wonder we sometimes got confused. The nodding heads around the table conveyed empathy, but also confirmed that everyone had noted my loss of face.

And so my downward slide continued. I knew I had to retire.

Dementia Field Notes

2-5-2011

During my going-away meeting with Gender Studies, the faculty gave me this journal. In it I'll report my descent into the post-cerebral realm for which I am headed. No whimpering, no whining, no despair. Just the facts.

3-3-2012

Saturday at the mall I performed the physical motions of shoplifting—walked out of Macy's with a pair of pants over my arm. I only noticed when I was inside Dillard's on the opposite side of the mall. I hurried back, ready to explain. There were no salespeople around, and no one noticed when I put them back.

3-8-2012

Took Bob and Diane to do their grocery shopping. (Been taking them since their son Bobbie took away Bob's keys after his stroke last year.) When we were done, I could not find my keys. The car doors were unlocked, the keys in the ignition. Returning home, I forgot to stop at Bob and Diane's and pulled into my driveway instead. Last time I took the old people shopping I did not notice the traffic light changing until Bea reminded me to go. She is eighty-six.

At home, too, my various slips proliferated. I spoke to my family and closest friends. "Senior moments," my peers knowingly declared. Even my then-twentysomething children, Marissa and Newton, assured me they, too, experienced similar lapses. As the incidents accumulated, though, my immediate family acknowledged that they noticed a change. As I approached my sixtieth birthday, they agreed that my deficits might be adding up to a diagnosable disease. I started considering making a doctor's appointment, my mother's mental unraveling never far from my mind.

On a February day in 1996, my mother, Susanna Catharina Steenekamp, was found wandering in her retirement center in Pretoria, South Africa, severely disoriented. A nurse led her from her stand-alone home to the sick bay, from where my sister booked her into the Little Company of Mary Hospital. When I arrived in her hospital room days later, she did not seem aware that I had come halfway across the globe. She did recognize me, however—my utterly proper mother introduced me to her nurse as "my daughter who writes *fuck*," an apparent reference to the language in my short story collection. Susanna also announced her every bodily function, saw angels, and poured water over herself "to bring down [her] temperature." With family, her loving disposition still came through, but with the black nurses her post-apartheid liberalism evaporated. She acted superior, entitled, rude.

Despite my mother's altered behavior, only my brother Boshoff, himself a doctor, mentioned dementia. In keeping with South African medical practice at the time of my mother's illness— proceedings that remain essentially unchanged as I write fifteen

years later—my siblings and I concurred with our mother's doctors that there was no need to push for an official diagnosis despite
the existence of tests. From this deliberately low-tech perspective,
Susanna was undergoing some form of mental diminishment characteristic of old age, in which her behavior would determine the
extent of assistance she would need. And that is how her second
childhood played out without a name.

As my mother attained a somewhat stable state after her breakdown, it was apparent that she would indeed need a high level of
care. My sister Lana put our mother's house up for sale, disposed
of her furniture, and found her a private room in an "old-age home"
that provided the twenty-four-hour care she needed. Surprising us
all, my mother came out of her deranged state within a year after
her dramatic collapse. When she "came to," my mother resolutely
refused to stay in a place that afforded her no freedom or privacy.
Lana reinstalled her in her house in the previous retirement center,
which fortunately had not yet been sold.

Back in her own home, however, Susanna frequently fell, often
injuring herself. She had trouble cooking—my sister Tertia once
discovered her eating meat that was still raw. Her nurses suspected
she was having a series of small strokes. After some months, it
became clear that her functionality had declined to a point where
she was incapable of living by herself, even with the help of a house
cleaner/companion twice a week, the watchful eye of the center's
staff, and the option to have three meals a day at the communal
dining room. Despite my mother's insistence that she was fine, our
family, led by Lana, moved her to an old-age home with levels of
care ranging from semi-independence to lockup. Susanna became
reconciled to the move when she found out that she would still be
able to visit neighbors and the library on her own.

Eight years after her initial collapse and facing rising costs, we
moved my then eighty-year-old mother to a more rural and cheaper,

yet excellent, care center in Cape Town under Tertia's care. She would spend her last two years in the landscape where she went to university and fell in love with my father, a fact she remembered even while forgetting her children's names.

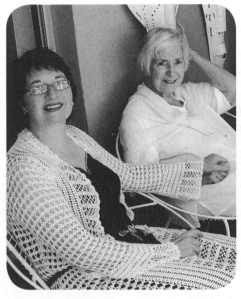

My mother, Susan Steenekamp, and I, shortly after her move to Cape Town in 2004. Our family held a Christmas gathering in Groot Brak, Western Cape, South Africa, at the vacation home of my sister and brother-in-law, Lana and Buzz Leuner.

My mother's deterioration had gone without a name. What, then, to do about my own unhinging? Even though much had been learned about dementia in the decade after my mother's death, all but the most occult sources concurred that there is ultimately no cure for dementia, or any other brain disorder with symptoms adding up to the gradual loss of intellectual function thereby "depriv[ing] sufferers from be[ing] able to think well enough to do normal activities, such as getting dressed or eating," "the ability to solve problems or control their emotions," as well as the adroitness to distinguish between things that are real and "things that are not there."

Despite the lack of anything approaching a "cure," there are medications thought to slow the progression of Alzheimer's and other dementias. However, my preliminary research confirmed what Peter and I had learned anecdotally: no existing medications could stave off the inevitable decline that catches up with even the most diligently monitored patient. We were afraid that the quest for diagnosis could trap us in what writer and physician Atul Gawande once described as "the unstoppable momentum of medical treatment." Still, we are both the kind of people who want to know, always drawn like moths toward enlightenment. Also, confirmation of our suspicions might help us prepare. If the unnamable loomed ahead, we could plan for expensive care, diminished quality of life, and a way to end my life at the right time.

I asked Peter to come along for that initial doctor's appointment in 2010. Our primary care doctor politely entertained our doubts about the value of diagnosis. She heard out our pontifications about what we regarded as a worthwhile quality of life, and let us stew our own way into following her suggestion that I have an MRI. The scan results showed "white matter lesions"—an indication of clogged microvessels that prevent blood from reaching nearby brain areas. Dr. Eborn confirmed the internet wisdom that microvascular dementia might benefit from cholesterol- and blood pressure–lowering medications to retard the clogging. However, a neurologist would first have to confirm a connection between my memory problems and the lesions.

One neurologist, one neuropsychologist, dozens of tests, and many hundreds of out-of-pocket dollars later, my neurologist uttered the d-word. She projected that two more neurological evaluations at two-year intervals would be needed before I would officially meet the criteria of dementia.

But in my heart I already knew: *I am dementing. I am dementing. I am dementing.*

Reflection on Dementia Field Notes of 8-11-2011 and 8-15-2011

Twice in August 2011, I jotted down notes in my journal about moments—possibly minutes—when I felt stark, staring mad. In the first entry, I tell about trying to rest in the afternoon and I keep on seeing columns of black and red Arial type scrolling on my eyelids.

A few days later, my entry was about sitting on my half of our two-seater La-Z-Boy reading *The Botany of Desire*. Soon after getting started, while paging over, I punched a hole in the page I had grabbed with the thumb and forefinger of my left hand. A few pages later, I apparently took up the page too roughly again, this time tearing out a corner piece.

Remembering the scrolling, I immediately thought that it was related to the book-ripping.

At the end of the week, however, while preparing our medications for the next week, Peter discovered that we had both forgotten to take our tablets the day before the scrolling. I knew that a sudden withdrawal of the drugs I take to counter my short-term-memory-loss-induced anxiety causes hallucinogenic effects. Thank goodness that turned out to be the cause—I thought I was getting even crazier.

It feels good to blame the lack of medication for the visual weirdness. However, I certainly have not forgotten my medication often enough to account for the fifteen months of weirdness I have so far recorded in my journal. While I do feel a bit crazy when I discover myself doing something unusual or illogical, I do not feel "mad" most of the time. Am I crazy like a fox? Or, maybe, Lewis Carroll's Cat?

Alice [asked the Cat]: "And how do you know that you're mad?"

"To begin with," said the Cat, "a dog's not mad. You grant that?"

"I suppose so," said Alice.

"Well, then," the Cat went on, "you see, a dog growls when it's angry, and wags its tail when it's pleased. Now I growl when I'm pleased, and wag my tail when I'm angry. Therefore I'm mad."

"I call it purring, not growling," said Alice.

"Call it what you like."

Or, maybe, like Frida Kahlo, I have resolved to turn "madness" into a desirable state? A curtain behind which "I could do whatever I liked"? Kahlo: I'd arrange flowers, all day long, I'd paint; pain, love and tenderness, I would laugh as much as I feel like at the stupidity of others, and they would all say: "Poor thing, she's crazy!"

Or, maybe, in this Don Quixote is my sage: When life itself seems lunatic, who knows where madness lies? Perhaps to be too practical is madness. To surrender dreams—this may be madness. Too much sanity may be madness—and maddest of all: to see life as it is, and not as it should be!

Whoever I decide to take as a role model for the lunacy that awaits me, I have already, like Charles Baudelaire, "felt the wind on the wing of madness."

Years before my mental disorientations had become a daily bother, in the days before Gender Studies when I was still employed in corporate America, I took a business trip to Raleigh, North Carolina, where Jacques,* a former computer designer colleague of Peter's from South Africa, then lived.

In South Africa, Peter and the man had sometimes gone to lunch or for a drink after work, but I had only met him and his wife—let's call them the Du Preez family—at company-sponsored social occasions. After both families emigrated to the United States, Peter and Jacques kept in touch, occasionally swapping stories of their experiences trying to settle into their respective states, and we learned more about his wife and family than we had known in our South African past.

After I landed in Raleigh, the Du Preezes duly picked me up at the hotel and took me to their home, where other South Africans would join us for dinner. After a nostalgia-triggering *braaivleis*, or barbecue, a friend of the Du Preezes', who had come to the *braaivleis* with a male partner, told us how he discovered he was gay. Let's call him Fanus.

Fanus grew up in the 1950s in a large, tough-love Afrikaner family that adhered to South Africa's most conservative social and political thinking. As far as he could remember, Fanus had always wanted to be a good person and adhered to the conservative norms of his family, church, and school. After high school he joined the army, where he first encountered the terms *homo* and *queer* and the many colorfully pejorative variations that proliferate in Afrikaans as well as in English, which served as the lingua franca of a country with eleven official languages. Since these terms came into Fanus's vocabulary sealed in a centuries-thick layer of negative associations, he had no doubt that moffies, skeefs, gayins, poofters,

---

* The names of places and people and other identifying information associated with this story have been changed at the request of the person whose story forms the core of my recollection and to whom I refer as Fanus.

pinks, fruits, dahlias, homos, queers, and those labeled with words he could not even bring himself to say were godless, unnatural people and the total opposite of the goodness he had pursued all his life. Accordingly, he joined his army buddies in taunting and terrorizing those unlucky few whose behavior or actions had marked them for torment in their heterosexual fellow soldiers' eyes.

After honorably completing his military service, Fanus started working in a business environment that was not quite as socially conservative as his hometown or the army. He made many friends, including a woman—say her name was Elsa—with whom he became very close. They spent a lot of time together. He started thinking about a future with her, a thought that made him extremely happy. She was the kind of woman his parents would love. She would be a good mother. He was young, however, and poor, and did not mention his dreams to her.

One day after work Fanus and Elsa were having a drink together, as they frequently did. Caught up in the warmth and comfort of their friendship, Fanus let slip the words "our future."

Elsa drew back, startled. After a few moments of trying to regain her composure, she leaned closer, took his hand in hers, and, in the gentlest, most caring voice, said, "Fanus, you and I have no future together. You are a homo."

When Fanus was telling this part of the story at the Du Preezes' party, his cup rattled in its saucer and he put it down on a side table. "When Elsa said that," he continued, "the lights of the world went out. An unspeakably foul, gray mist stretched all around me. My life had no shape, it was barren."

Everyone at the barbecue became totally quiet. Fanus went on. "After a long, long time," he said, "the lights of the world came back on. Color seeped back into my life. Objects fell into their contours like figures developing on a Polaroid. I felt bloated with relief, a helium balloon." As joy spread from his mouth to his eyes, he riffed on his own metaphor. "A homo balloon. I was a homo. I am a homo."

During the days following my neurologist's pronunciation of my brain's fate, snatches from the evening at the Du Preezes' home in Raleigh bubbled into my consciousness like unrelated happenings in a dream. With the only tool at my disposal being a sidelong familiarity with Freud's nineteenth-century dream analysis, I was unable to decipher the significance of this in relation to anything going on in my life at the time. After months of thinking about it, however, it occurred to me that what I remembered had everything to do with the sense that my self-perception, my identity indeed, had been undergoing a monumental change from the moment my neurologist reported my test results. The memory that eventually emerged from the shenanigans of my subconscious not surprisingly turned out to be Fanus's story—or, more accurately, the core of Fanus's story, which, as I learned when I tracked Fanus down, had in the interim been encrusted with details from coming-out stories I had heard from other friends or gender studies students.

In the days after my neurologist gave a name to what was wrong with me, the separate circles in which I had kept the images of myself as *a woman who lives and dies by her rationality* and that of my mother after her illness as *a Dickensian madwoman* gradually began to overlap like the intersection of a Venn diagram. Within that convergence, I came out to myself in tones that sounded believable to my skeptical ears: *I am dementing. I am dementing. I am dementing.*

Chapter Two

Quantum Puff Adders and Fractional Memories

I DAILY CONTINUE TO LURCH into that "strange Country," with "all Things new, and unknown about," a territory demarcated by the intersections of my past, present, and future selves. In the past—really until I was in my late fifties—I took my good memory for granted in the way that one does other privileges into which one is born: my middle-class existence, my good health, my entitlements as a white person in South Africa and the United States. In reflective moments I was guiltily grateful for these gifts, but in my daily life I did not stop to consider them. They were just part of who I was.

In the present—from the time my short-term memory started to fail—I frequently am bewildered about why, where, and who I am: What was the goal that had bounced me out of bed and sent me outside to stare at the garage door? What store am I in? Who is this person I call "I" who feels so lost in a world that, all of a sudden, seems to tilt from its axis?

My perplexity in the present also reaches back into the past. If, at the end of every day when we sit down with a glass of wine to watch a video while holding hands, Peter and I have the same argument about whether we have finished watching our previous night's film (I swear we haven't, whereas Peter is equally certain that we have and he reminds me of the ending and I concede that he was right), what truth value does my vivid, thirty-year-old memory of our seventeenth wedding anniversary merit? And yet, it plays like a video on my closed eyelids: Peter at home with Newton; I in a motel room in Vernal, Utah, with my girlfriends Kathy and Anne, chaperoning our elementary-school daughters on a trip to the state-level Olympics of the Mind competition, which, the next morning, they won. And what about the Technicolor veracity of sixty-year-ago scenes from my childhood about my life on the Steenekamp family farm in South Africa?

I was four years old in 1953 when we moved eight hundred miles northeast from Cape Town to the Transvaal, a region as different and as distant from my birthplace as Chicago is from a farm in Kansas. The idea was that my father, Boshoff, would help my grandfather on the family farm. In retrospect, I realize that my father—who had lived away from the farm from age thirteen until after he had completed his degree at Wits University and worked as an engineer for five years—had reverted to the role of an apprentice, albeit a voluntary one. His older brother, Koot, who had also returned to farming after living away for a dozen years during which he completed his engineering education, had already been inducted into the mysteries of farming by their father. Koot had completed his apprenticeship some years before our move and had been farming his portion on his own for some years. He would be my father's mentor. My father would start his training by working his own land. Once the farm started yielding an income, he would build a house on his portion and move our family there. In the meantime, my parents, siblings, and I lived with our grandparents in the Old House. From there my father drove the seven miles to the fields and back every day, often more than once.

Counting my father, three of the five Steenekamp siblings lived on the farm at this time, and soon a fourth—an aunt returning from England—would join us, too. Our aunts, uncles, and their families—including nine cousins from age four down to newborns—all lived within walking distance or a short drive away. By the time I was seven years old, my parents had built our own house on the portion of the farm that my father inherited, a plot of about a hundred imperial acres, or *morgen*, Dutch for "morning." A morgen is approximately the amount of land tillable by one man behind an ox in the morning hours of a day, equivalent to about three-quarters of an American football field. Parts of our hundred morgen had been plowed and planted in former years, but, according to the known history of the area, no white settlers had ever lived on the land before. If any of the Bafokeng, the original Tswana-speaking inhabitants of the area, were still living on our land when the Steenekamps started farming there in 1838, I was not aware of it.

Our Steenekamp forebears joined other Voortrekkers, or First-Leavers, who had had it up to their eyebrows with the British rulers, who had won the colony from Holland in 1806 during the Napoleonic wars.

My Voortrekker ancestors joined a party of other disgruntled farmers, loading their ox wagons and setting out northward, together with hundreds of other family parties, on the Groot Trek, or Great Migration, into the wild interior. Along the way, they battled indigenous peoples for land and passage with their superior weapons—guns against assegais, clubs, and sharpened sticks. An ancestor on my grandmother's side was six years old when Sotho warriors, ancestors of the Transvaal Bafokeng, attacked her party's encampment at the Bushman River on February 17, 1838. From her hiding place amid the reeds on the marshy riverbank, she watched as her parents and siblings were speared and clubbed to death. According to family legend—and a photo of a grim-faced woman in a bonnet in the Old House—she wore her trauma like a badge of distinction. As family legend has it, she never smiled again until her death.

The Voortrekker Steenekamps settled in the Rustenburg district on land then still occupied by the Bafokeng, who, by then, had fallen on hard times and welcomed the newcomers as a source of employment. They named their farm Beestekraal, Cattle Corral. The farm my grandfather acquired during the 1930s and my father inherited in the 1950s was twenty-six miles from the Voortrekker homestead.

Our new house was as basic for 1956 as Beestekraal's first dwelling of reeds plastered with clay was for the 1840s. Our home consisted of a spare, L-shaped outbuilding that was supposed to be converted to storage rooms after our "real" house was built. The roof was of corrugated iron, the floor concrete. By my mother's insistence, our house had a ceiling and larger windows than the peepholes customary for a storeroom. Just as well, because my father's ship never came in, and the building of our house never proceeded beyond the foundations, which were dug and poured soon after the completion of the storerooms. The setting of our temporary house, at least, was spectacular: from every vantage point, one could see all the way to the horizon that, to the north and east, was demarcated by low ridges known as the "black hillocks" and, to the south and west, by the Magaliesberg range—mountainous parentheses that encircled our home. Inspired by the spectacular view, my mother named our farm Die Kraaines, or the Crow's Nest.

As was then customary when a patriarch divided his land among his children, my father also "inherited" two black laborers whose families had been employed by the Steenekamps for generations. Ou

Isak and Ou Naald were indentured servants of sorts. Although the *Ou* in their names means *Old* and is nominally a form of respect, we white people often acted disrespectfully toward them. For example, I remember when one of our aunts, exasperated that Ou Naald, who was deaf and whose back was turned when she shouted an instruction, did not react, she hurled the soapy water from a jug she was washing onto his back.

How my mother—a former social worker who had worked with nonwhite people—and my father—a mining refrigeration engineer who had gone to the politically liberal (that is, anti-racial-discrimination) University of the Witwatersrand—experienced the farm's raw version of the government's 1949 institution of apartheid, I can only vicariously imagine. In truth, my parents' daily worries were probably subsumed by the uncertainty about ever recouping the enormous loan they had procured from the Land Bank to pay for everything from farm equipment to the laborers' first year's pay. However, my father's big dreams must have carried him through, as evidenced by the many enthusiastic discussions he had with his brother, who had left mechanical engineering to farm, about modernizing tobacco and wheat farming by employing scientific analyses, methods, and reasoning.

The farm was harder for my mother, I believe, whose entire life since teendom was geared to leaving the hardscrabble country existence she knew only too well from growing up on a Kalahari sheep farm. Moreover, she had to contend with the Steenekamp women of my grandparents' and her own generation, who looked on her as a foreigner with strange ideas about everything from raising children to serving beets raw. And then there was the loss of amenities: in Cape Town we had electricity; on the farm candles and lamps and a coal stove for hot water sufficed. (Our cooking stove mercifully ran on natural gas.)

My mother had dreams, too: she regarded the farm as a canvas for her creative spirit. As soon as we moved in, she planted a willow tree at the back of our house, and a bougainvillea against the stark, whitewashed wall by the front door. Visitors driving up on our dirt road were greeted by a flower garden and the beginnings of a lawn in front of our house. Just inside our other "front door" that opened into the long hallway that led to our bedrooms, she placed a wall hanging made out of a hessian bag emptied of seed wheat and encouraged us to pin plants, flowers, insect carcasses, and mouse skeletons on it for display. In the absence of fresh flowers for the combined living-dining room, she made an arrangement the size of my four-year-old brother out of dried branches, pods, veld greenery, and other found objects that struck her fancy. She encouraged us to follow her example and put together our own creations for our bedrooms.

Oblivious of the political, financial, and technological constraints on our parents, my siblings and I embraced our new life with gusto. Our cousins formed a ready-made peer group whose games of building houses out of sticks, sliding down the grassy earthen dam wall in a cardboard box, and robbing birds' nests of eggs and fledglings were far more gripping than the in-retrospect mundane hide-and-seek games we used to play with our Cape Town neighbor kids across a span of two measly city backyards.

By the time we moved to Die Kraaines, there were four of us, five-year-old Lana and I—then seven years old—having been joined by two brothers, Klasie, four years old, and Carel, almost two. The brothers shared a room, we sisters another. When another brother and sister arrived a few years later, they moved in, too, maintaining the gender lines. When I was fifteen years old and my boyfriend visited from Johannesburg, he bunked with the boys as well.

When Carel was still a toddler, we oldest three set out on what we considered hair-raising adventures facilitated by the merciful paucity of adult supervision in those days. When he was a bit older, Carel was a regular member of our expeditions. Our exploits included the discovery of a cave in a rocky outcrop two miles from our house into which we would let ourselves down with ropes we carried from home, and where, after a disappointingly short drop, we would come upon the bones of a jackal still bristling with a few patches of fur. At the same rocky outcrop, our six-year-old cousin Katrientjie once accidentally put her hand on the miniature paper-lantern hive of a swarm of wasps. After being stung multiple times, she lost her grip on the rock face, tumbled six feet to the ground, and broke her arm, a string of events that necessitated eight-year-old Lana and six-year-old Klasie, fast runners, to race back for help, while ten-year-old me took charge on the injury site. Until help arrived, I held Katrientjie's head on my lap, spoke whatever reassurances I could muster into her ear, and squeezed juice from an orange on her lips and into her mouth with the notion that the sweetness would stop her from fading in and out of consciousness.

The *shaba* on the *pap*, or the gravy on the grits, of our adventures, though, if measured by the frequency of its retelling, must have been the slaughter of thirty-nine deadly puff adders. The puff adder is a venomous viper found almost everywhere on the African continent. Its venom causes severe cell destruction that leads to extreme pain and swelling followed by widespread necrosis and, within twelve to twenty-four hours, death. Today a person bitten by a puff adder can be treated with a life-saving antivenom, as long as it is administered within a few hours after the strike. Without treatment, which is still not widely available in less populated areas, a victim will likely die within a day. Even people treated with antivenom often lose one or more limbs to gangrene, depending on the speed of treatment, the quantity of venom delivered, and the site of the strike.

We started learning about snakes as soon as we moved into the Old House. Whenever one of our family members or a farm laborer killed a snake, the person who killed it would give us a lesson over the mashed-up remains. The curled-up one that my aunt found sunning itself on the back step was a black mamba, even though it was actually brown—it got its name from the black color inside its mouth. The skinny one that surprised my cousin Hendrik by dangling from a branch overhead while we were climbing the fig tree and was killed by my grandmother's gardener with a rake was a green *boomslang*, or tree snake—there were brown ones, too. The shiny coppery one that lifted the front of its body as high as the bucket by the water tank and spread the skin behind its head into a hood was a cobra. The only snake we saw alive was a *molslang*, or mole snake, and since it wasn't venomous we were allowed to pet its shiny black scales and crowbar head.

We never laid eyes on the snake that I remember best from the time we still lived in the Old House. One morning one of my grandfather's laborers brought his toddler daughter to the house for help. She had been bitten by a puff adder the day before. Despite the *sangoma's muti*, the traditional healer's medicine, the little girl's arm and hand were swollen beyond recognition. Though it looked terribly sore, she did not even cry. Her eyes were open, but she did not flick away the flies sucking the bubbled spit from the corners of her mouth. My grandfather drove her to the doctor, but she never came back. She died before the doctor could even send her to the hospital in Brits that served the black population.

In the days that followed, the grownups would tell us to put on our shoes before we left the house. They proceeded with a warning to look out for puff adders. My father gave us a dramatic explanation that almost caused me to stay inside permanently. "Puff adders are everywhere," he said in his ghost story voice, "but they're lazy and won't come after you. So it's up to you not to scare one or step on one. They're difficult to see—they blend in with the shadows under the trees. Keep your eyes open for the shine of snakeskin. If the puff adder notices you first—it smells you when it flicks its tongue—you'll recognize what it is from the way it coils into an S and pulls up its head this high." He made a wave for the coils and drew a line with his finger just below my knee. "You'll hear it suck air to inflate its head and hiss it out again." My father mimed the snake's puffy head with his cheeks and imitated the sound with a spit-spattering hiss. "If that happens, run home as fast as you can to get me or Mamma or any other adult so we can kill it."

On the day of the record-breaking killing, though, vipers were far from my mind. I was eleven and just about to go off to boarding school. My oldest brother, Klasie, now seven, and I were out in the *veld* together, about two hundred yards from home, test driving the stilts we had made that morning by nailing jam cans onto thick sticks of wood, when we spotted, protruding from a gap the size of a pencil box in a four-foot-tall pile of rocks, a bulge of snakeskin. We could see the gleam of black chevrons on a grayish brown background.

When we noticed a snake in the rock pile, Klasie and I wasted no time trying to identify it. We hopped down from our stilts and ran home, yelling the whole time for our father and Ou Isak. Pa, we realized when we got back home, was out in the tobacco fields. Ma was home, though, and hurried back to the rock pile with us to have a look.

After verifying that the snake was real and, indeed, enormous, Ma took action. She told us to keep watching the snake, which hadn't moved at all since we first noticed it, and went home to find Ou Isak so that he could get a shovel and a pick-axe and guard the snake with us while she called my father's older brother, Oom Koot, who had a gun. Despite the growing crowd of spectators, the snake did not change its position. Eventually Oom Koot arrived and identified the snake as a puff adder. His wife, Tannie Wientjie, who had come along for the excitement, did not really want to look at the snake, but could not resist a peek through her fingers. "It would make a lovely handbag," she said. By that time Pa had joined us. With all the bystanders clumped together on some wide flat rocks out of the bullet's range, Oom Koot took his shot.

The instant the bullet penetrated the snake, its skin burst open and out came what seemed like hundreds of foot-long baby snakes that scambled down the rocks and onto the trampled grass around the pile. The ground was alive with sinuous, wriggly miniature puff adders. Mixed in with the living ones, pieces of those hit by the bullet were still curling and twisting. We were farm people used to killing animals, so most of us sprang into action. Everyone— except Tannie Wientjie, my mother (who was pregnant with the baby that would be Boshoff), and I (who had killed a few things before but had decided I didn't like it, or was I scared?)—grabbed a stick, a large stone, or one of Ou Isak's farming implements and started killing baby snakes. Those of the participants who had sticks flipped the baby snakes from the grass over to the flat rocks, and those with stones, picks, or spades bashed or chopped them until they were dead. Over the killers' laughs and squeals and yells and the gritty, percussive scrape of tools on rock, the nonpartici-pants shouted warnings to be careful, since even newborn puff adders are venomous enough to kill an adult human being.

When the snake slaughter at the rock pile was over, we lined up what was left of the mother as well as the dead baby snakes. The killing ground was littered with snake pieces. We laid them on the ground, end-to-end to approximate the length of a whole one. After the reconstruction, we counted thirty-eight babies. The mother made thirty-nine. No one had a camera, except Oom Kris-jan, who was working at the car repair shop and filling station he owned and was therefore not available to snap the scene. By the end of the day the snakes were no more. Ou Isak had taken the mother to the tobacco drying barns to roast and had burned the not-worth-eating babies, so neither skins nor skeletons survived.

The story, however, lives on and has entered the lore of a fourth generation in our clan, which is now without our parents but has grown to almost forty people by the addition of the six siblings' husbands, wives, children, and grandchildren. Our children and their cousins claim that the number of snakes has multiplied every time they have heard the story told. However, we siblings who were *there* stand by our count of thirty-nine, even if a handful of these were composites.

Fluit, fluit, my storie is uit—shout, shout, my story is out.

Dementia Field Notes

8-24-2011

I could not combine the up and sideways movements of our bathroom tap to make cold water come out. Instead fetched cold water from the kitchen in the plastic jug.

5-16-2012

At La Frontera I was unable to interpret the beer stein the server put before me. I knew it was a beer stein, but couldn't absorb the fact that it was upside down. I saw it as right side up with a tight-fitting glass lid, which I tried to take off. I asked Peter how to get it off, and he turned the glass around. Then I understood. We were with friends.

5-24-2012

Here at the vacation house in Zion National Park I have trouble reading the diagram for the stove plates. I meant to switch on the kettle and instead switched on the pan of oil. Fortunately Newton saw it and prevented a disaster.

After my retirement in August 2011, I needed almost six months before I felt ready for what I had looked forward to for most of my working life: preparing an almost-done novel for publication and completing a second one, into which I had already poured years of time and research. However, my last years at Gender Studies had left me fearful that I might not be able to edit a three-hundred-page novel and resume another; at work, writing had come to drain my mental energy to the point where I had none left for my family or home life.

Just about every aspect of my university job had involved writing. The program emails, office circulars, meeting reports, letters of recommendation, and other official letters had been quite doable just about up to the time of my retirement—they were relatively short, self-contained pieces. However, longer research-based documents—which I used to love—had become very difficult. After thinking about my retirement writing projects for a month or two, I decided against revising my books-in-progress until I had a better sense of whether research-based writing and editing for my own purposes would be less anxiety-provoking than it had been at work. I instead started writing an essay about the changes with which I am struggling as the result of my encroaching dementia. While I had learned a bit about dementia in the lead-up to my diagnosis, I did not possess enough knowledge of the brain and how it works to write the kind of essay I liked writing, namely part personal and part research-driven. I would have to educate myself. By then I had been recovering from my work-related stress and exhaustion for half a year. I felt it was at least worth a try to see if my head would work any better than before.

It did. The time I had taken off after retirement, as well as the fact that my new writing was on a topic I had chosen and about which I was passionate, resulted in my focus being somewhat sharper, though I was still not able to do without laborious notetaking. The pages grew in slow motion, but grow they did. When the first essay was done, I wrote another. For reasons I did not then understand, the project was becoming increasingly important to me. With the hindsight of four years, I now think of it as Gerda's Last Stand.

About four chapters in—the chapters you encounter here are not in the order I originally wrote them—my better-than-expected progress became its own puzzle. Looking back at the work I had completed, I asked myself, "How come I can still write? Could I be faking dementia?" Since the indignities accumulating in my daily activities, which I had been recording in my journal, as well as the conversation-inhibiting lacunae in my speech are classic markers of early dementia, the discrepancy between those failures and my preserved writing ability are part of my story, too. I wanted to understand why. Here is my report, the results of my self-imposed, self-designed course in introductory neuroscience.

Is It Possible for Dementia Patients Who Have Lost Their Independence in the Performance of Activities of Daily Living (ADLs) to Retain Deeply Engrained Knowledge Structures and/or Intellectual Skills?

This report consists of five parts: (1) What is memory and how does it relate to "truth"?; (2) Enquiry into the truth of "The Tale of the Thirty-Nine Puff Adders"; (3) Why can I still write, and are there any other dementia sufferers who similarly lose their abilities in some areas of their life while retaining them in others?; (4) Post-hoc email commentary from the two snake-killing eyewitnesses and one earwitness; (5) Post-post-hoc email commentary from the senior snake-killing eyewitness and the not-yet-born earwitness.

Part I
What is memory and how does it relate to "truth"?

Research sources: Peer-reviewed neuroscientific journal articles available on the internet, popular science magazines, and self-observation.

Results: When we use the term *memory*, we usually have long-term memory in mind. However, events stored in our long-term memory will already have passed through two earlier stages of memory making: first, the sensory stage, which consists of registering a perception and keeping it in short-term memory long enough to judge it as a keeper or a fly-by-nighter; and second, retrieval of all associations related to the perception that have earlier been stored in long-term memory, combining those and the new perception into a revamped information package, testing the worthiness of the updated batch, and—should the package pass the "value added" test—laying it down in the brain areas available for long-term memory, or memory that often lasts years or a lifetime.

As its name implies, short-term memory is not long for this world. Accordingly, the brain real estate available for keeping it around is limited: enough for retaining only four to six chunks of information for about twenty or thirty seconds. A memory's life span can be somewhat extended if the perception lends itself to being broken into chunks and you repeat the chunks in your head—a phone number, for example—thereby resetting your short-term memory clock. However, not all perceptions can easily be chunked. Even a basic perception generates a vast amount of information: cognitive representations, such as concepts or previous experiences; sensory data, such as visual images, sounds, touch, smell, or a combination of these; and emotions ranging from disgust to pride to shame to happiness. Information of this complexity will be lost after about half a minute unless the perception seems important enough to warrant further attention.

The part of my memory that is most affected by my dementia is the part of short-term memory known as *working memory*, or the ability to hold a small amount of information in my head while I manipulate it. This morning, I got dressed and picked earrings studded with pink diamanté to wear with my outfit. I used the mirror in our closet to put them on. After I had gone to the upstairs bathroom to put on makeup, I noticed that I had lost one of the earrings. I backtracked down the stairs and to the bedroom looking for it. It lay on the shelf by the mirror in the closet together with the winged nut that secures it behind the ear. My attention had drifted after I had put the first one on, and I left the second one behind. In the same way, when I take out the garbage in the midst of cooking dinner, I could a minute later be watering my new plants outside while the broccoli boils dry. I have changed from an efficient and goal-directed person to someone who drifts from task to task, sometimes striking a blank between deciding to fetch the milk for my coffee and reaching the fridge one step away. In situations like this, realizing that I can't remember what I was up to, I stop in my tracks, wring my hands Lady Macbeth–like, and ask myself, "What am I trying to do?"

Long- and short-term memory use the same storage areas, which are scattered throughout the brain. Cognitive information such as words, concepts, and numbers is stored in the gray matter of the frontal cortex, the area in charge of the so-called higher brain functions. Sights, sounds, and touch also have their places in the frontal cortex. Smell, however, is stored in the olfactory bulb, which is located in a crucial part of the brain's apparatus for transforming short-term memory to mid- or long-term, the *limbic system*.

The limbic system's primary function is to manage our hormones, and thereby direct our emotions and feelings, which proves to be an indispensable part of a well-functioning memory system: the stronger the emotion accompanying a perception, the more likely it is to become a vivid long-term memory.

Limbic System

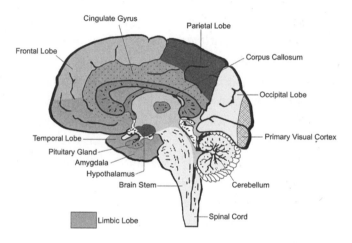

The crucial role of emotional significance in forming memories is a recent discovery, achieved in the last decade as a result of new neuroscientific instruments such as functional magnetic resonance imaging (fMRI) that enable live observation of the brain as it performs memory-making or -retrieval tasks. That there can be no memory without emotion "is a radical departure from the traditional perspective, which used to regard emotion as the antagonist of reason." The insight has led to a paradigm shift in contemporary brain science: "We simply cannot understand thought without understanding emotion."

To dig a bit deeper, I extended my exploration to find out what is happening on the level of my neurons, or cells in the brain, spinal column, and nerves that are specialized to transmit nerve impulses. What is going awry with the way my memories are laid down, recalled, and refiled? Some interesting insights come from the study of disorders that are in a sense the opposite of forgetting. In post-traumatic stress disorder, or PTSD, the sufferer is precluded from living a normal life by the inability to forget a horrific memory. The explanation, as with forgetting, lies in the cellular bricks and mortar of the brain.

Electrical circuits that support the making, recalling, and modulation of long-term memory function like a grid of power lines across a vast landscape. The "wires" consist of neurons that have been made sensitive to each other so that when one fires, all the others go off at the same time. These neurons have been fitted with parts that make it easier "to pass on their electrical excitement." When the limbic system decides that a memory is worth keeping, it releases hormones that trigger DNA along the activated circuit to manufacture protein building blocks. Those blocks physically strengthen the connections between neurons by shaping themselves into additional receptors or neurotransmitters, thereby reinforcing the brain's capacity to retain memory over time.

Once a pathway for long-term memory has been laid down, there is no guarantee that it will survive. It may end up being only a mid-term memory unless it is constantly maintained. Since typical neuron proteins start breaking down within as little as two weeks after being formed, "every long-term memory is always on the verge of vanishing." The continuous repair of disintegrating neurons is known as *reconsolidation*.

Psychiatrists have for decades used the principle that memory circuits must be reconsolidated to help people move on from a traumatic past. Through trial and error they discovered a class of drugs that was successful in taking the edge off horrific memories, thereby allowing more new pathways to be formed through suggestion or techniques of positive reinforcement. Successfully treated patients remember the traumatic experience, but have shed the fear, anger, and other negative emotions associated with it.

Functional imaging research has now revealed that the class of drugs that had success in treating trauma-related disorders all have in common the ability to trigger the production of an enzyme, PKMzeta, that *blocks* maintenance proteins to the areas where emotions are stored while the sufferer recalls the traumatic event. This means that the signal-strengthening parts of the old circuit are not replaced, and the memory fades.

The discovery that "memories are not formed and then pristinely maintained," as neuroscientists used to think, but rather "formed and then rebuilt every time they're accessed" has far-reaching implications: every time we think about the past "we are delicately transforming its cellular representation in the brain, changing its underlying neural circuitry." So, a memory is changed every time it is remembered.

These findings upend the model of memory (still) held by most people, namely that memory "works like a video camera, accurately recording the events we see and hear so that we can review and inspect them later." It raises questions whose answers may have far-reaching consequences. Given our contrary new understanding of memory recall, what is the status of our legal system's reliance on the veracity of eyewitness testimony? Closer to home, what is the veracity of my cross-my-heart-and-hope-to-die puff adder story?

Part II
Enquiry into the truth of "The Tale of the Thirty-Nine Puff Adders"

Sources of information: email interviews with two eyewitnesses and one earwitness to the snake killing.

Results: Since no childhood photographs or family letters about the puff adder incident are available, I tasked my siblings, both the eyewitnesses and the ones who have heard the story told all their lives, to check my version of what happened.

Our conversation was launched via email on September 27, 2013, the day after my sixty-fourth birthday. All my siblings, now in their fifties and sixties, were included. I began by recapping the story as I remembered it, accounting for the possibility that we might have counted half-snakes as wholes. I requested, in Afrikaans, that "those who had already been born and could walk and attended the snake killing" send me their variations of the story. I ended my email by passing on a conceptual schema in relation to the story that my middle brother had mentioned during a phone conversation he and I had had about my little project: "Carel came up with a lovely name for a story with so many disputable facts: 'Quantum Puff Adders.' Please cast your quantum in the snakeskin purse."

The replies came fast and furious.

Klasie, 9-27-2013:

If we counted halves, there would have been 19½ whole ones. No, there were 39 little ones. Your description of the rocks where the snake was shot sounds odd to me. The largest rock was drilled and blasted with dynamite, why and what for I don't know.

Carel, 9-27-2013:

I suspect that Gerda is conflating two snake episodes; fusing fractional memories into integral recollection—in this instance puff adder/makoppa fusion.

The reality, as Klasie and I concur, involves him, myself and I think Duard or Willie urinating on the pile of rock debris when the cry of "slaaaaaang" resulted in a frantic and wholly undignified scramble past and through the karee and wag-'n-bietjie bushes on the dam wall to inform what we at the time considered to be a responsible adult. Oom Koot arrived first but unfortunately unarmed. Characteristically unflustered in the way that distinguished him from his younger brother,* he kept an eye on the snake while the 12-gauge shotgun was being fetched from I think Martiens Barnard or a neighbor further down that road. In the re-telling, Oom Koot was blowing pipe smoke at the snake— presumably to keep it enthralled while awaiting its demise.

From that point my recollection roughly concurs with Gerda's.

Klasie, 9-27-2013:

Yes, Carel's story is how I remember it too. I don't remember the spade and Isak. Does that come from another story? If Duard were there, his father would surely have arrived with many guns.

Carel, 9-27-2013:

A merely honest person can't deny another's clear recollections; a tactful and magnanimous one is required for that. The physical evidence for the puff-adder story was destroyed in a tobacco-drying furnace almost 50 years ago—all that remains are those fragile palimpsests we call memories.

I have little ego vested in this scenario, but I entertain the notion to start doubting my own recollection, if only for rhetorical purposes.

I am going to make an annotated map of the events and send it out.

---

* My father, Boshoff Steenekamp.

Carel sent out the Google map below, whereupon Klasie responded with his own map in Excel titled "Farm by My Mem." Below, I place the maps one beneath the other.

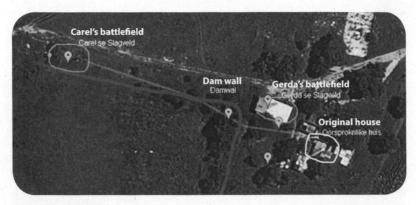

Carel's Google Map

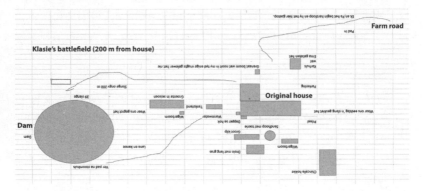

Klasie's Excel Map: "Farm by My Mem." I flipped Klasie's map horizontally and vertically so that its orientation would be similar to Carel's, hence the upside-down, mirror-image original labels.

Together with his map, Carel also sent a diagram he had drawn with a note explaining "that [it] gives more detail about my memories of the slaughter." He titled the drawing "Carel se Slagveld," or

"Carel's Battlefield." (Just as well drawing talent was not a prerequisite for Carel's success as a computer entrepreneur ☺.)

Carel's battlefield

Boshoff (who had not yet been born by the time of the snake incident), 9-27-2013:

This is history and because it's history, I know best. I cannot recall the incident at all, but I have heard the story repeatedly from several different observers. Accordingly, I have the advantage that my personal observations are not influencing the objectivity of others.

There were 39 snakes. Pa himself shot the snake with his .22 pistol.

> "History is that certainty produced at the point where the imperfections of memory meet the inadequacies of documentation."
>
> —JULIAN BARNES, *THE SENSE OF AN ENDING*

Gerda, 9-27-2013:

Boshoff, I am happy that your objective history has now placed a firearm in our own Pa's hands, albeit one with a short barrel. What is history if it is not patriarchal?

Carel, 10-1-2013, subject line "Laaste skoot na die pofadder," or "Last potshot at the puff adder":

Klasie, I'm impressed with your map. One problem is that the dam was not round, but rectangular, as the blue line [on my map] shows.

Two items remain before I can clock out with my puff adder memories intact and unassailable: 1), Question for Klasie: who were there when the snake was spotted the first time? 2), I will undertake an in situ inspection for terrain corroboration. Yours in Aspergers.*

Gerda, 10-1-2013:

Carel, your terrain corroboration will be worth exactly as much as the number of siblings you take along (obligatory smiley face here: ☺). What point is there to being correct when no one is there to whom you can say, "I told you so?" .

Klasie, when I mentally plot my site onto yours, they are an exact fit. Does that mean you and I actually agree on something in the universe? Carel, on your map the killing field is too far from the house. I guess that is a vote of two against one!

In your battlefield sketch, however, my scene looks remarkably the same as yours, Carel. That makes a fifty-fifty split. However, there were definitely not as many as 20 onlookers. Our whole

---

* Several members of our family are on the autism spectrum, fortunately at the high-functioning end. Some of us are self-diagnosed, while others have been identified as such by the psychiatric establishment.

family was there, Oom Koot and Tannie Wientjie, Ou Isak, but no contingent of black children. The invisibility of black people under apartheid may have skewed my memory in this regard.

Conclusion: As the conversation continued, each person's memory was jogged by other versions in such a way that we reached a near-consensus on key aspects of the event: the approximate location of the place of slaughter, the live emergence of the baby snakes, number of snakes, and the use of a firearm as well as ad hoc tools found on the site to kill the baby snakes. While we all stick to some of the impressions with which we came to the discussion, no one believes the others are flat-out lying.

Our family's experience in comparing individual memories is congruent to my finding that the brain refreshes the "truth" every time you retell it. In relation to the memoirist's assertion that a story is true, I conclude that the strongest claim she can make about a story from her past, especially those to whom there are no eyewitnesses, is that a narrative is true "as remembered and affirmed by the storyteller."*

Part III
Why can I still write, and are there any other dementia sufferers who similarly lose their abilities in some areas of their life while retaining them in others?

Information sources: Peer-reviewed neuroscientific journal articles, popular science magazines, interviews with health professionals, and self-observation.

Results: I am not the only person who appears to be "faking"! For example, a counselor friend tells of a retired philosophy professor

---

* *Moth Radio Hour*'s disclaimer before their weekly show in which participants tell stories from their lives, rehearsed but without notes.

from her alma mater who can no longer bathe, dress, or feed himself, but directs canonical philosophy discussions with visiting former colleagues. A sprinkling of peer-reviewed neurological research, too, reports the "unexpected preservation of a cognitive function in individuals with dementia": in the neurology journal *Brain*, for example, researchers Julia Hailstone and Rohani Omar present the case of a sixty-four-year-old semiprofessional harpsichordist with a non-Alzheimer's dementia who "had virtually no comprehension of oral or written language," "was mute," and did not understand the functions "of objects such as a corkscrew and a tuning fork," but nevertheless demonstrated "the motor skills required in playing [his] instrument," "the visuoperceptual skills required to read scores," and "the cognitive skills involved in interpreting symbolic notation" as attested by his performance of "technically demanding, structurally complex compositions in an expressive manner."

During my search for accounts of the experience of dementia, I also came upon David Shenk's best seller on Alzheimer's, *The Forgetting*. During his research Shenk discovered Morris Friedell, a sociology professor diagnosed at age fifty-nine, whose final year of teaching, four years before his diagnosis, sounds uncannily like mine.

> ...he began to have trouble remembering what his students said in class. Later, he couldn't remember a conversation he'd just had with his mother. At the neuropsychologist's office, he couldn't tell the doctor about a movie he'd seen just the night before. They ran the usual tests. He got a perfect score on the MMSE [Mini Mental State Exam, a test done in the doctor's office which includes determining the patient's orientation to time, ability to repeat three unrelated words right after the tester has said them, naming objects, and reading and following instructions]. On the brain scans he didn't fare so well.

After a year of long-distance interaction, Shenk met Friedell in person at an Alzheimer's conference at New York University, where Friedell did a poster presentation titled "Potential for Rehabilitation in Alzheimer's." During lunch with Shenk the next day, Friedell explained that for him rehabilitation no longer means "intensive rehab, in the spirit of what knee and hip surgery patients go through," but rather "minimizing and slowing the cognitive loss by adapting to it." His method includes performing an extremely simple task "just to get into a confidence mind-set," and from there taking on the challenge "to solve problems in new, simpler ways."

After lunch, Friedell asked Shenk if they had "ever spoken before today."

So, it seems that dementia can sometimes go like this: persons having spent a lifetime mastering particular knowledge structures and intellectual skills may retain access to this expertise even after becoming utterly dependent in daily activities. I want to believe this will be my story, too. But in truth writing is getting slower and harder: the six chapters I have so far completed, excluding the current one—which, I imagine, will be my last one—took three and a half years of many eight-hour days, reams of notes, endless thesaurus-mining, scissors-and-tape cutting and pasting to figure out how a single comprehensive piece might come together, and the tough-love edits of writer friends Shen Christenson and Kirstin Scott.

Dementia can also go like this: a person having spent a lifetime mastering particular knowledge structures and intellectual skills—a well-educated person, in other words—may for a while use a "greater 'thinking power'" to compensate for the disease in its early stage. However, as *MailOnline* reporter Jenny Hope brought to light, research done at the Albert Einstein College of Medicine of Yeshiva University shows that once university graduates' dementia becomes evident, they "suffer a memory decline that is fifty percent faster than someone with a minimal education."

My father: Your education is something you can always fall back on.

My mother: Dreams are easy, but the gander lays the egg.

Einstein: The faster you go, the shorter you are.

Doña Quixote: Finally, from so little sleeping and so much reading, her brain dried up and she went completely out of her mind.

Part IV
Post-hoc email commentary from the two snake-killing eyewitnesses and one earwitness

Gerda, 10-1-2013:

Boshoff, the new Julian Barnes quote you passed on from Daleen really puts its metaphorical finger on the combination of "facts" and the embellishment of memory: "And the longer life goes on, the fewer are those around to challenge our account, to remind us that our life is not our life, merely the story we have told about our life."

My skepticism about religion started in earnest when I first read the biblical exegesis that gives the dates of composition of the various sections of the Bible and discovered that all of the books were post-hoc accounts, removed from the events by as little as 60–70 years and as much as several centuries. So how about the Exodus 7 snake story:

[10] Aaron cast down his rod before Pharaoh...and it became a serpent.

[11] Then Pharaoh called the magicians of Egypt and they did in like manner with their enchantments.

[12] But Aaron's rod swallowed up their rods.

Carel, after studying your map, I saw that you had become smarter and smarter overnight and your memory better and better. Your snake story has now gobbled up all of the stories the rest of us have told. Unlike Pharaoh who hardened his heart at the display of God's power, I am hearkening onto our Carel-Moses to part the waters of the Sterkstroom when we all join you in the in situ inspection! (o.s.f.h. ☺)

Carel, 10-1-2013:

I am in my noppies (fat dumb and happy) with the "emergent Truth" and look forward to our en masse bethinking of our testimony at the altar of the Snake.

Part V
Post-post-hoc email commentary from the senior snake-killing eyewitness and the not-yet-born earwitness

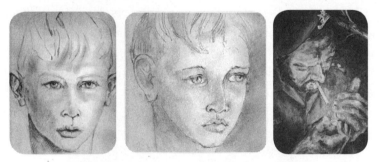

Klasie, 8 years old. Carel, 6 years old.* Boshoff in his 30s, self-portrait[†]

Gerda, 9-2-2014, subject line "Die pofadder het weer uit die dode opgestaan," or "The puff adder has once again arisen from the dead":

Working on my book. The now documented story is MY truth, since if we go by seniority, I likely remember best, given that

---

* My school friend Erna Schutte, now Buber-deVilliers Schutte, sketched my two older brothers during a visit to our farm.
† Boshoff's self-portrait, *Boetman*, 2000.

memory is strongly associated with words and I had many more words at eleven than you, Klasie and Carel, at seven and five.

Long live the puff adder!

End of Research Report.

Coda to Research Report

Part VI
Frangible memories

Email, Gerda to American family, 10-9-2014:

My beloved brother Klasie died today at the age of sixty years, two weeks after being diagnosed with non-Hodgkins lymphoma. His daughter Vida called at 3 am our time to tell us. He died with his wife, daughters and stepdaughters, and grandchildren at his side. Tertia and Mickey were there too, they also called us. He died on the living room couch, where he had spent the last days of his life with kids clambering over him during the gaps when morphine dulled his pain.

Klasie, my big brother, I've loved you since you were my little brother and love you now.

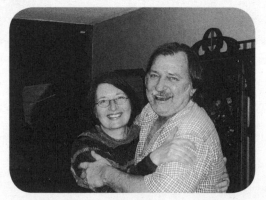

Klasie and Gerda in South Africa, 2002

It seems to me that the discrepancies among witnesses to the killing of the thirty-nine puff adders could be subsumed under the current neurological model for memory—every time you recollect a memory in spoken or written narrative, or merely think of it in private, it gets changed and reconsolidated. However, other attempts to check the veracity of stories I reported in my journal have not gone so well.

Item: A friend, who mercifully is now an even better friend, was "aghast, horrified, actually" about my retelling of his coming-out story he had told me decades earlier. When I looked into the matter, I found out I had conflated his story with that of another person in a way that made him seem much more naïve than he had been about his sexuality.

Item: More than a year before my diagnosis, I accidentally gave a doll from my children's baby days to my son Newton and his wife Cheryl's daughter, Aliya. I was convinced the anatomically correct, newborn-sized boy doll, named Bossie for my father, was the one we had bought for Newton when he was born so as to parallel the anatomically correct, newborn-sized girl doll that we had earlier given to Marissa. I was "aghast, horrified, actually," when my children corrected me: both dolls belonged to Marissa. Moreover, Bossie was not just any doll, but rather newborn Newton's gift to his sister at the moment he first met her when she came to the hospital, so that, as the parenting book suggested, she would have her own new baby and not feel left out because of her infant brother.* How could I have forgotten an event into which so much planning had gone? As a photo shows, I had even placed Bossie next to Newton in the infant crib on wheels in which the nurse had brought

---

* The hopes we had been led to harbor for the efficacy of the gesture in preventing all sibling rivalry, not surprisingly, turned out to have been fictional.

him to my room from the nursery where he had been for observation so that he could give it to his big sister. Moreover, this event
had happened only thirty-five or so years earlier. What did that
mean about my memory of events going fifty, sixty years back?
To correct my doll blunder, I sheepishly explained to two-year-old
Aliya that Ouma—my grandchildren's name for me—had made a
mistake and asked that she give the wrongly gifted doll back. Fortunately that turned out great, since Aliya had decided that boy
dolls are no fun because their clothes are not pretty.

Given that my memory already has a record as long as my pro-
verbial arm, how can I possibly vouch for the truth of the stories I
tell? Truth is, I can't. It is little comfort that, according to leading
neuroscientists, nobody—not even the most honest writer who also
happens to have an expansively documented past—can swear that
everything she tells is "exactly how it happened." Be that as it may,
I have less confidence—and rightly so—in affirming the "this-is-
exactly-how-it-happened" status of my recollections than I imagine most other memoirists do. My fading memory is a fact that,
whether I fess up or not, figures into every story I tell.

As the seventeenth-century translator of *Don Quixote* asserts
about Cervantes's protagonist, though, my lies, too, "are not of the
highly imaginative sort that liars in fiction commonly indulge in;
like Falstaff's, they resemble the father that begets them; they are
simple, homely, plump lies; plain working lies, in short."

If you know that you will get things wrong, why, then, write in
the memoir format, a genre in which writers are always in danger
of being accused of "nudging" the truth, making things up or—
Oprah forbid—completely fictionalizing?

I write memoir for selfish reasons: it is a way, accessible to me
and preferable to playing memory games on Lumosity, to flesh out
my shrinking self with former selves.

I write to remember, to inhabit, for a while, my earliest self, an entity I describe by appropriating Carel's portrayal of *his* first self in his poem "Heimat," a self "formed by straight tobacco rows… / where the earth was deep, rich, moist and black." Unlike the spoiler snake of the Bible, the Snake with a capital S from my childhood is not an instrument of banishment from paradise, but rather a means of re-entry into the wonderland in which my soul unfolded before the "withered crops, pestilence and winter's cold" had "conspired to my father's broken dreams." Once my mind "had warmed / to treasure islands," I probed the world beyond our encirclement of mountains and greedily made it mine, grasped time in my two-fisted clutch and pressed it to my heart.

I write to admit, from my crone's nest atop the "strange Country" with "all Things new, and unknown about" in which I am growing old, a sky-high bird's-eye confessional, stripped of lattices and screens and open to the world—I write to admit that the more the world around me confuses me, the better it feels to escape to that patch of earth, "deep, rich, moist and black," where my desires are still "bounded by the mountains, and if they ever stray, it's only to contemplate the beauty of the heavens, the steps by which the soul is shown the way to its first dwelling place."

I write to internalize a Law of Nature, a fiat not subject to human understanding or memory, a truth I intuited as a child witnessing wriggly life without number turn to thirty-nine unmoving columns of death, a truth I assimilated intellectually as a young woman studying quantum physics, a truth I must now embrace with my fate-battered psyche: time's arrow points only one way—forward.

I write to embrace my place in the cycle of the generations. My body, my brain, my cells—all subject to the Second Law of

Thermodynamics: the entropy, or disorder, of this, my closed system, always increases, until its parts no longer cohere and again return to the elements that birthed them.

Deep, rich, moist and black.

I write, in other words, so I won't die of Truth.

Chapter Three

The Grammar of the Disappearing Self

Even now, as dementia wreaks its havoc on my short-term recall, memories from my childhood in South Africa persist in vivid detail.

One Sunday afternoon, when the world of the family farm was still new, my father took me along when he went out to see how the tobacco seedlings were coming along. Four years old and filled with self-importance, I climbed into the passenger seat of our second-hand blue Willys and my father drove off along the two-track road with the high grass *middelmannetjie*, or central ridge, that scraped the bottom of the car and that the recent to and fro of farm machinery had carved from the veld. After a short drive, past the tobacco kilns, past the water pump, we stopped on the road.

Pappa lifted me onto his lap so I could see out the window. I remember his eyes through his glasses looked as big as an owl monkey's. Curls of smoke from his cigarette perfumed my hair. Beyond the blue of the car door, Bible-black soil stretched bumpily toward the horizon. About twenty steps into the choppy blackness, a white patch of ground winked in the sunshine. It was rounded at the top like a small dune, or a high-water dam some big girls had built on the beach back in Cape Town. Already feeling the *kielie-kielie* of the sand between my toes, I said, "I want to go play." Pappa opened the door and looped me out onto the grass beside the wheel tracks.

Feeling the grass prickle against my tender feet, I held on to Pappa's fuzzy leg. In Cape Town we had worn shoes and socks all the time, but I was determined to get tough like my cousins and had peeled off my shoes the minute we got out of church that morning. As we climbed in the car after the sermon, Mamma had, as always, insisted that my sister and I follow her example in staying in our church clothes until after our midday dinner—she had given up on the shoes and socks—but she said nothing when Pappa stripped off his tie and jacket even before we had left the parking lot. At home, he had immediately changed his suit pants for everyday khaki shorts. In the lands that day, as he stood beanstalk-tall beside me, the only sign of his church attendance that remained were his black deacon shoes and socks. It would take many years before I would add together his resistance to church clothes with his scientific world view to understand that he was an atheist. Oblivious of such matters on that Sunday, I scooched up the skirt of my pink dress and tucked it into the leg holes of my panties. Gingerly I stepped out on the sharp-edged clods with wheat stalks sticking up from them, yellow and brown.

"Where are you going, Gertjie?" Pappa called.

"I'm going to play in the sand," I said.

"What sand?" Pappa asked.

"Over there," I explained, pointing toward the white beach I saw in the distance.

My father dropped to his haunches, wrapped his arms around me, and stood up. Pointing to the white shape, he explained that it was actually a plot of germination beds that had been seeded with tobacco a few days earlier and covered with strips of cheesecloth suspended by wires. He had spoken about germination and had even put a pinch of the flyspeck seeds on my palm. "Berrinkies," he reminded me.

In an instant, the whole scene snapped into comprehension. I recalled the soft bed of cheesecloth that fell in folds to the floor by the dining room table where Mamma's Singer would whir for a whole day as she stitched lengths of the white fabric together. In the living room, my sister Lana and I would stake out our separate territories in the unworked fabric, only flying out of our soft nests when Mamma called for help. I would flap over to the Singer so Mamma could arrange a l-o-o-o-ng veil of fabric on my head, and I would spread my arms like wings and glide outside to the far edge of the prickly brown lawn, where I let the veil slide off me like a cloud leaving the moon. In the meantime, Lana would clamp the next piece of fabric in her pointy-armed wing and drag it to where Mamma was rubbing her wrists before again cranking the Singer's handle.

That day in the lands as I lurched in Pappa's arms high above the black turf toward the seedbeds, his breath in my ear and his heart boxing with mine, awe spiraled around me like wisps of smoke: A word can do that! A word can change sand into cloth!

Berrinkies.

The astonishingly prolific British author Iris Murdoch published twenty-six novels in her lifetime. Additionally, her oeuvre includes five books on philosophical issues, six plays, and two volumes of poetry. Murdoch's prose vacillates between astutely observed and hilariously bizarre, the whole brimming with dark humor and unpredictable plot twists. Her storytelling strips her stiff-upper-lipped characters of their veneer of civility. As she peels the onion of their selves layer by layer, she reveals a hollow core echoing with yet more language.

In her fifteenth novel, *The Black Prince*, Murdoch depicts the reverberating core of the self as an instrument of redemption, the only route to divinity, albeit one purified of religion. Under her pen redemption comes about through words: my self is only what I say, and only by opening myself to the pain of my words can I attain the redemptive pleasure of claiming to be a self at all.

Bradley Pearson, *The Black Prince*'s narrator-protagonist, explains to Julian, the twenty-year-old woman with whom he is in love, why *Hamlet* is his favorite work of art. "*Hamlet* is words," Bradley says, "and so is Hamlet...He is the god's flayed victim dancing the dance of creation." The god is Shakespeare himself, who created Hamlet and then emptied out the prince's self by—in Murdoch's image—peeling his living body out of his skin. When Julian asks whether Shakespeare isn't then turning Hamlet's pain onto himself, Bradley responds,

> Of course...But...because love here has invented language as if for the first time, he can change pain into pure poetry... He [transforms] the purification of speech...[into] something comic...Shakespeare cries out in agony, he writhes, he dances, he laughs, he shrieks, and he makes us laugh and shriek ourselves out of hell...What redeems us is that speech is ultimately divine.

Murdoch's own relation to words, speech, writing, stands testament to her conviction that there is no self without language, no route to "ultimate divinity" without the mediating power of words. Predictably, then, her writing is characterized by a rich and imaginatively deployed vocabulary. However, in Murdoch's later novels the kinkily erudite lexicon that used to be an essential part of her identity becomes progressively depleted.

Upon the 1995 publication of *Jackson's Dilemma*, which would be her last novel, Murdoch's critics and admirers alike were struck not only by the work's impoverished vocabulary, but also its lack of coherence and other oddities. As Susan Eilenberg put it in the *London Review of Books*, gone were "the perfection of tone, the witty throwaway symmetries of accident and insight, the artfully balanced...rhythms and geometries of passion and form" that had for so long characterized Murdoch's writing. These trademarks of mastery had been replaced with "prosiness...didacticism, and... reliance on whimsy, allegory and magic," which Eilenberg found tedious. Following the launch of *Jackson's Dilemma*, Murdoch's audiences at public appearances noticed that she often appeared bewildered. In 1997 a medical diagnosis confirmed what some had begun to fear: the grande dame of British literature, then seventy-seven, had Alzheimer's.

With revisionary hindsight, everyone from linguists to neuro-scientists to her own husband found in Murdoch's past behavior and writings harbingers of the dementia that would completely erase her identity—and indeed her life—in the short span of two years. Her husband, John Bayley, traced journal entries back to 1993 that struck him as out of character. While Murdoch had based the very possibility of a relationship with Bayley on his unqualified respect for her private self-sufficiency—a stipulation that even required him to condone her affairs that spanned their forty-five-year marriage—in her final years Murdoch declared a growing emotional dependence on him that implied the fracturing, even the disintegration, of her formerly impenetrable self. Affectionately referring to him as Puss, she writes, "My friends, my friends, I say to the teacups and spoons. Such intense love for Puss—more and more." After Murdoch's death, Bayley applies the idiosyncratic wisdom of the poet A. D. Hope to their last years together by saying that he and Iris had moved "closer and closer apart."

Bayley found Murdoch's journal entries from 1993, two years before *Jackson's Dilemma* was published, unambiguously troubling.

"Find difficulty in thinking and writing," she wrote. "Be brave." Four years later, during the year Murdoch was diagnosed with Alzheimer's, she composed a note that was downright ominous. "My dear," she wrote, "I am now going away for some time. I hope you will be well…" She set aside the sheet, took up a second one, and wrote, "My dear, I am now going away for some time. I hope you will be well." A third sheet consisted of pen marks that did not add up to any intelligible lines.

As Murdoch's illness continued to crumble away her language and reason, she gradually abandoned attempts to write. Soon sense departed from her speech as well—except to him who loved her deepest and longest. There came a day when Iris laid her hand on Puss's knee and said, "Susten poujin drom love poujin? Poujin susten?" Bayley needed no more help than her hand gentling his cheek to distill from this jumble the grammar of love.

Like all white farm children in South Africa during the 1950s, I knew that I would be going to boarding school once I reached my teens. Since I started school at five and subsequently skipped a grade, I was two years younger than my academic peers. For me, therefore, emancipation from the relatively untrammeled part of childhood came three months after my eleventh birthday, in January 1961.

In South Africa of the 1950s and 1960s it was a cultural mandate that white children should succeed academically because it was our patriotic duty to advance our race on the Dark Continent. My parents' focus on education went far beyond this: they valued intellectual development as a good in itself, as the very beacon of honorable personhood. Even though each successive year of drought or hail or infestation of cutworm plunged my father deeper into debt with the Land Bank, and even though my siblings and I wore homemade clothes and the hand-me-downs of our better-off cousins, my parents drilled us in our times tables and my father coached us in the arithmetic, algebra, and the science of the everyday world at every opportune moment from breakfast to bedtime. We started learning English before we even started school through my mother's daily after-dinner reading from children's classics mail-ordered from overseas, including standbys like *White Fang, Robinson Crusoe,* and *Treasure Island,* as well as finds like Enid Blyton's Adventure Series, which were instrumental in preparing me for boarding school. (It would be many years before it would occur to me that none of this anticipation would have featured in the dreams of the black children on our farm, upon whom I had for the past six years looked down from my seat on the bus as they ran to school on the shoulder of the road, their lower limbs grayed by the dust their feet raised from the road's narrow shoulder.)

Even though my boarding school would have hardly any resemblance to the one in Blyton's novels, in January 1961 I confidently set out for Rustenburg Hoërskool. My whole family made the drive—about an hour by car from our farm—to deliver me to the complex of buildings constituting the school hostel (what Americans would call a dormitory), where I would live for nine months out of the year.

My family accompanied me into the annex—a temporary building of the kind today being dismantled with asbestos caution methods—where an overflow of two dozen standard sixes and a prefect would live in two identical sleeping halls, or dormitories, under the supervision of a "housefather" who occupied an apartment at the end of the hallway with his family. Once we had located my bed, it was time for my family to leave. Since, in my intellectually snobbish family, my attainment of boarding school was by fiat an occasion of pride, there were no tears. Within the span of five on-the-mouth kisses, I was alone with my suitcase. I set out the school clothes that I helped my mother sew over Christmas on the light blue bedspread bearing the letters TOD/TED (Trans-vaal Onderwys Departement/Transvaal Education Department): two dark green *gyms*, or pinafore dresses (with matching panties—bloomers, rather); five white blouses; and a church dress, also white.

My dormitory was almost as large as our storeroom house. The space was divided in half by a double row of army-green metal cab-inets, arranged back-to-back. On each side of the divider, a black metal cot, head end abutting the opposite wall, mapped one-to-one onto each cabinet. Six girls were assigned to each side. At the bed next to mine, a yet unnamed roommate was just finishing her unpacking. The girl's cabinet doors were open, revealing a closet with eighteen inches of hanging space on one side and eighteen inches of shelving on the other—an entire closet that did not have to be shared with anyone else!

I savored the luxury of placing my treasures, each according to its kind, in the first roomy space I could ever claim as my own. Already I was gluttonously attached to this territory, where my possessions would stay as I had decreed, where the vanity case where I magpied away my special things—the powder-puff-soft tuft of rabbit fur I pulled off a fence barb; the three spotted guinea fowl feathers I salvaged from a spot next to the coal heaps behind the tobacco kiln where our laborers plucked wild birds to roast in the always-lit fire; my pads and belt for when I would get my first period; and the lemon facial astringent I had made from a recipe in *Die Sarie*, an Afrikaans woman's magazine—would not be raided by a covetous or curious sibling.

If the thirteen-year-old girls on my side of the dormitory were surprised to find a flat-chested and periodless eleven-year-old among them, they showed it only by taking a patronizing stance toward the "Little One." It would be many years before I would fully comprehend the extraordinariness of my teenage roommates' indulgence during that year. How naïve, decades later, was my expectation as an immigrant mother that my own children, accents obvious, would be embraced by their peers as they set forth into the foreign territory of American teendom.

About a month into the term, our first "hostel weekend" arrived, one of the twice-per-quarter paroles when we could go home. My father picked me up on Friday afternoon. During the hour-long drive home, he quizzed me about algebra, beaming proudly when I reported that our class had not yet worked up to the difficulty of the equations he had already taught me to solve. When his inquisition turned to Latin, he surprised me with an off-color joke—albeit by the standards of the day—that he had apparently been hoarding since his own high school Latin years. "Translate *apis potand abigone*," he said. Desperate not to let him down, I talked out my meager vocabulary: *apis*, didn't that have something to do with bees? Could *potand* be an odd conjugation of *potere*, which means "to be able to do." *Abigone?* The ablative absolute of a verb I hadn't yet encountered? The more I speculated, the more my father guffawed, setting off his smoker's cough so vehemently that we momentarily swerved into the oncoming traffic. After regaining his grip on the steering wheel, he spilled out the solution. "Punctuate it like this," he said. *"A pis pot and a big one."* We laughed until Pa's cough nearly took us off the road.

At home, the lamps were lit, the table set, the food ready to serve. Although it was our house servant* Anna's night off, she stayed until I got there to show me her new baby, a girl named Kagiso. My siblings seemed a bit shy at first and passed me the gravy and the butter as if I were a guest. By the end of the meal, though, things were back to normal. My brothers' protests against

---

* It is of course no longer politically correct to say "servant" (even in South Africa), but this is how we then referred to a job now titled "domestic assistant."

bathing drowned out the news on my father's radio, and Lana and I got into a row that repaired our attenuated sister bond. In the morning, demonstrating a complete lack of appreciation for the fact that I never got to sleep in on Saturdays at school, my mother woke me before the grid of window sun even got to my feet so I could hem a set of flannel nightwear for our new little brother or sister, who was due to arrive six weeks later.

When I rejoined my roommates on Sunday night at the dormitory, some girls were crying, but that ended as soon as we started exchanging goodies from home. It felt a little bit lonely after all the noisy family togetherness, but it also felt good to be back in an ordered space where bells chimed the days into predictable chunks, meals automatically appeared in the dining hall, and every building of the hostel uncannily went quiet for study. I loved being able to do my homework in the neon glow of overhead lights, without the acrid smell of moths immolating themselves in the lantern flame.

That night, I was borne into sleep on a wave of belonging, my worlds having been sewn together like the pieces of a baby's night wrap. I was shocked when, within days, unpredictable spasms of homesickness cramped my insides. Sometimes there was a reason, such as the day a sudden rainstorm struck while our whole hostel, two girls abreast, was snaking up the hill to school. With squeals and shrieks our formation splintered, every girl for herself, even the prefects. Never having been a good sprinter, I fell behind. When I tried to catch up, I slipped, skinning my knee. As I hobbled through the gate after the last of the other girls had already made it inside, I felt more alone than ever before in my life.

Though the shame of being left behind wore off somewhat as the days passed, icy shards of longing still impaled my innards at unexpected moments. While I did feel loved by my roommates, I also yearned for someone I could really talk to, like my friend from back home, Jacoba, who was the only person I knew who read the same books as me and loved to discuss them. The girls in my sleeping hall did not read any books other than those required for school or talk about anything other than the upcoming interschool sports day when the whole school would go by train to Pretoria. Jacoba attended one of the most prestigious schools in the country, Pretoria's Afrikaanse Hoër Meisieskool. Though only seventy miles from Rustenburg, Pretoria might as well have been Pluto as far as Jacoba and I were concerned: neither of our families had the means for frivolous travel, and, besides, Jacoba's home weekends fell at different times in the school term than mine.

As I lay awake listening to the slumbering breaths from the beds beside me, I imagined Jacoba in her hostel, luxuriating in a warm bath, since surely her hostel had enough hot water for even the standard sixes; snuggling with a book among her down puffy pillows and plump comforter until she was sleepy, and then clicking off her own light, which was right next to her bed.

Eventually, my thoughts would return to óur farm, the lands, the night sky where my father—that magnificent atheist in deacon's clothing—and I would track the planets, locate newly rising constellations, and during the giddy twenty-one days of Sputnik, try to spot it as the satellite whirled cheekily around Earth, at one hour and thirteen minute intervals, until it sank below our horizon.

I thought, too, of the noisy bustle inside our house after my mother had given her last warning for us all to come in: my father tickling five-year-old Carel and seven-year-old Klasie off the couch so he could claim his seat by the radio for the seven o'clock news; my mother threatening from the kitchen that someone had better light the lamps and set the table; my jealousy of the praise my mother heaped on Lana for not only having lit the lamps but also washing their glass globes; and after dinner, my father again claiming the couch, grinding out his *stompie* in the overflowing ashtray on the side table by the radio, and lighting another cigarette before scrutinizing the newspaper. I thought of my brother Klasie's yells when I accidentally tunneled into the quick beneath his bark-like soles while needling out a thorn; after my mother took her place in the wicker chair, we children jockeying for space on the nearby blanket we named Wollie; and my mother's head bobbing in and out of sight behind the book she was reading out loud, translating the story for us, sentence by sentence, from English into Afrikaans as it unfolded.

Calling home to alleviate my homesickness was not an option. The pay phone in the main hall was reserved for emergencies. Trying to recall my family members' faces made it even worse—in place of their images appeared instead a desolate wasteland swirling with snow, like the one the girl Gerda from Hans Christian Andersen's fairytale had to cross to save her dearest friend, the boy Kay, after the Snow Queen had spirited away his memory and frozen his heart. Nothing could save him but Gerda's tears, rivers of warmth that melted the frozen crust that trapped his heart and rekindled his memory, upon which they sped home on a fleet-footed steed—what Gerda, then, would weep hot tears for me?

In *Elegy for Iris*, John Bayley writes, "I was far too preoccupied at the time to think of such parallels, but it was like living in a fairy story—the kind with sinister overtones and not always a happy ending—in which a young man loves a beautiful maiden who returns his love but is always disappearing into some unknown and mysterious world, about which she will reveal nothing."

During my research on dementia, I read a review of Bayley's memoir that cited this baneful observation about his and Iris Murdoch's relationship. Reading it out of context, I assumed that it referred to the period when Alzheimer's was encroaching on the couple's lives. I was surprised to discover that the passage instead describes the early years of their marriage. For years after their marriage, by his own admission Bayley grappled with his wife's need to seal off areas of her life from him. In the "fairy story" chapter, Bayley tells an anecdote that illustrates his early awareness that their relationship was going to be challenging. His insight came the first time he and Murdoch went dancing: when they stepped onto the floor, filled with Bayley's friends and acquaintances, hardly anyone was dancing, chatting loudly over the music instead. After Bayley introduced his date, Murdoch got along so swimmingly with her new friends that Bayley, a bit miffed, invited her to dance. When they moved to the music, "there seemed to be no correlation among the different parts of [their] bodies." Leaving Bayley to his "unconfident...hops," Murdoch broke away to execute her own "ungainly...arm twirling and arabesques." When, seconds later, she inadvertently bumped into a couple dancing together, the man smiled and, breaking away from his partner, took Murdoch in a dance embrace. "She melted into him," Bayley writes, "and the pair swung off in perfect unison."

After submitting to many even-harder-to-stomach instances of Murdoch's "going away"—including her multiple affairs—Bayley launched an effort to cultivate a similar "apartness" for himself, a state of mind in which he, like Iris, would be "hermetically sealed." His "solitudes," however, would not include sexual or romantic infidelity. A few years after the start of his quest, he claimed that his sealed-off realms had become pleasurable, "a little like having a walk by oneself and knowing that tomorrow, or soon, one would be sharing it again with the other, or, equally perhaps, again having it alone."

To some of Bayley's readers and critics, Bayley's professed acceptance of Murdoch's need for extreme privacy rings hollow. They perceive his exposure in his memoir of intimate details of her mental infirmity—while she was still living, albeit in a state where his revelations could not hurt her—as a betrayal. A revelation they find offensive, for example, is his description of a trip to the bathroom where, after she'd had a bowel movement, he "wiped her bottom and scrubbed her hands and her brown fingernails," soiled as a result of her own efforts to clean herself. Critic Carol Sarler interprets Bayley's "demeaning, diminishing, reducing and insulting" of Murdoch as a form of Schadenfreude by a man who had been overshadowed by a "hugely achieving" woman. Other critics explain Bayley's unflattering disclosures about Murdoch as a phenomenon sometimes found in memoir or other biographical writing about the dead.

Like Bayley, I myself tell tales out of school in order to expose the unsavory realities of dementia, and I come down on the side of those who believe that through his shocking disclosures combined with his unfailing care "Bayley demonstrates how love still thrives in such uncompromising familiarity [and that] this book reveals itself as one brave enough to face such ambivalence as well as the horror of dementia."

The last of my three brothers, Hennie-Boshoff, was born in 1961 on big brother Klasie's eighth birthday, May 16. There was still almost a month to go before my next weekend home. My father had driven my mother to the maternity home in Rustenburg near my school for the birth, which, as was customary in the 1960s, he did not attend. Once my brother had been delivered, he went home to take care of the other children. When my father visited her the next day, he got the housefather's permission for me to see my mother and the baby. Hennie-Boshoff's mouthful of name was intended to distinguish him from my father, who went by Boshoff. The baby wriggled in my arms, contorting his face as if practicing for laughing, crying, being surprised. I only visited once, though my mother stayed three days. On the third day my father fetched her and the baby home.

A week or so later, I was lying on my bed during the mandatory rest hour after school. I was practicing Latin declensions when I noticed through the open curtains that the tree to which I sometimes fled to read my book was starting to turn the orangey-brown of autumn. The curtains were breathing in and out unevenly in the slightly moving air. I squinted to make out the red TOD/TEDs stamped across the surface. With my eyes scrunched up, the folds in the corner of my eye became the dunes that edged the white Cape Town beach. In an instant, I was four years old again, huddled in my father's arms at the edge of the lands. *Berrinkies*, my lips said. *Berrinkies*.

When the study bell rang, I made no move to get up. Piekie, my window-side neighbor, came over and nudged me. "Study hour," she said. Her words made my father, the farm, the dunes vanish. I wasn't angry. I just felt flat. I knew I could get up if I put my mind to it, go to my desk, say hello to Rina, a prefect with whom I shared a desk, and spend the rest of the hour reading the chapter we were assigned from *De Kleine Maja*.* Something unyielding inside me, though, made me just stare slightly to the side of Piekie's nose as if I were looking right through her.

Piekie tried a few more times to get me to respond, but her coaxing just reminded me of how, back home, my mother sometimes sweet-talked me into reading a story to my brothers, but I would usually refuse because my own book was so much more interesting. I now felt bad that I hadn't listened to my mother, hadn't been kind to my brothers. I wished it was my mother by my side now, not Piekie, asking me so nicely. If only she were here, I would get up immediately, would apologize for having been selfish. Was I being selfish now? Was I even here? Who was that girl lying on the bed, her tongue heavy, her breath too thin to speak? Why was she being so naughty?

---

* A Dutch book that was part of our Afrikaans curriculum.

When Piekie called Rina, I was scared that she would immediately detect my misbehavior. However, though she was a prefect,
Rina did not see into my sinner's soul. And so my muteness continued through the housefather's scrutiny, and that of Matron, the hostel nurse, who had been summoned from the main building. After
sitting me up so gently that tears spilled onto my cheeks, Matron
gripped me by the elbow and led me over to the main building. My
heart womped noisily in my chest as I lay between the sick room's
stiff sheets, my gaze fixed on the halo of gray hair surrounding
Matron's nurse cap. She took my temperature and applied her
stethoscope to my rib cage. Even those instruments did not reg-
ister the deception of my heart, the perdition of my soul. Instead,
Matron had the kitchen send me soup and called my parents.

In the morning, I sat waiting on the chair next to the bed in the
same clothes I had changed into after school the day before. My
school bag was at my feet. Rina had brought it over with my tooth-
brush and washcloth stuffed among the books. It felt very wrong
not to thank her. After she left, I listened and listened for the roar
of our Willys in the parking lot. I attempted to read one of the
books from my bag, *De Kleine Maja*. I tried my voice by reading a
sentence out loud: it croaked in the silence of the sick room, but it
was there. I should have tried harder last night, I thought. I was
deeply ashamed of having been naughty. My parents would be so
disappointed.

I did not breathe while a three-headed silhouette approached the
bed. When Matron stepped aside, I saw it was *them*. I was over-
joyed to see that they had brought the baby. I did not run toward
them, though I lifted my face for a kiss. When they asked how I felt,
I still did not meet their eyes, just said, *"Goed."* Matron left, and Ma
and Pa proceeded to ask more questions. I looked them in the face
and answered clearly. I couldn't explain it, I said, but I just could
not talk. A knowing look played between them. When my mother

put Hennie-Boshoff in my arms and let me carry him to the car, I knew I was forgiven. On the way home, and during all four days of my unscheduled hostel weekend, we never spoke about my bad behavior at all.

This episode taught me another astonishing thing about words: if you could not say them, your outside self disappeared. Inside you became the eerie cave on the farm, its rank interior littered with the bones of dead animals. Yet you dared not open your mouth, lest your raveling self burst out like thirty-eight baby puff adders only to be chopped into little pieces that could never again be put together into perfect little shiny, wriggly lives.

It would be many years before I would learn about dissociative mental disorders. The description of depersonalization in the *Diagnostic and Statistical Manual of Mental Disorders IV* sounds eerily like the detachment I experienced during what I have always before thought of as a voluntary episode. It was only when my children had reached the age at which I went to boarding school that I understood how the defeated slump of a girl tucking *De Kleine Maja* into a book bag would have placed her on a terrifying trajectory in a parent's heart. The forgiveness I read on my parents' faces was more likely an expression of dread—they were, I now think, wondering whether the intellect on which they were banking my future could harbor the seeds of its own destruction.

Iris Murdoch was notoriously private. She rarely gave interviews pertaining to anything other than her literary work, and then only with her guard firmly up. Her reluctance to share her life was not restricted to journalists. Anyone who aspired to be close to her had to respect her need for privacy as the sine qua non of the relationship. After meeting Bayley, Murdoch made it clear from the beginning that he would be no exception. She intended to go on functioning as an utterly self-contained person exactly as before, keeping areas of her life in compartments hermetically sealed even to him. Her need for what he refers to as "apartness" did not preclude a devotion to Bayley that he would eventually conceive of as far more lasting, generous, and encompassing than the fleeting passion shared with the men and women with whom she engaged in affairs. The marriage that resulted was, to put it mildly, unconventional. In Bayley she found the rare individual who would accept her demands, though it did not come to him easily. In *Elegy for Iris*, the first book in a trilogy Bayley wrote about his life with Murdoch, he describes how he overcame his unease about her lovers. "In early days," he writes, "I always thought it would be vulgar— as well as not my place—to give any indications of jealousy, but she knew when it was there, and she soothed it just by being the self she always was with me, which I soon knew to be wholly and entirely different from any way that she was with other people."

Given Murdoch's well-known desire for privacy, her apparent concession to turn her journals and manuscripts over to Bayley for publication was a radical departure in her behavior. Did she give up her privacy because her fame had made it impossible to keep news of her illness from the public? Had the dementia already changed her identity or eroded her self-confidence, thereby engendering a reliance on Bayley that brooked no resistance? However it came about, through Bayley's publication of a chapter of *Elegy for Iris* in the *New Yorker* in July 1998 and the completed book a few months later, outsiders gained unprecedented access to Murdoch's "case" even before her death in February 1999.

After Murdoch's death and the confirmation of her Alzheimer's through autopsy, Dr. Peter Garrard, a neuroscientist at the University College London and the Medical Research Council's Cognition and Brain Sciences Unit, was drawn to her as an ideal object of study: could her abundantly documented mental life yield clues of a cognitive decline not yet measurable by clinical tools such as the MMSE

(Mini-Mental State Examination), a questionnaire used by researchers and medical professionals to screen for dementia? Since Murdoch wrote only in longhand, made few revisions to her manuscripts, and seldom allowed publishers to make any changes at all, her manuscripts, Garrard wrote, "offer[ed] a unique opportunity to explore the effects of the early stages of Alzheimer's disease on spontaneous writing." Should the in-text harbingers of insidious cognitive decline that Garrard hypothesized be confirmed, the oeuvres of other novelists, as well as collections of letters, diaries, or blogs of people later diagnosed with dementia, would become a valuable resource for study on how, in Garrard's words, "the vast, structured network of information that endows objects and words with meaning" breaks down.

Garrard and his team analyzed the manuscripts of three novels that trisect the span of Murdoch's career: her first published work, *Under the Net* (1954); a novel written during her prime, *The Sea, the Sea* (1978); and her final novel, *Jackson's Dilemma* (1995), written before she showed any signs of cognitive decline. They compared characteristics such as grammar, narrative structure, vocabulary range, word types (i.e., nouns, verbs, conjunctions, pronouns, and other word categories), and the rate at which previously unused words are introduced.

Garrard's results reveal that Murdoch's linguistic creativity dwindled markedly over an almost twenty-year period, that is, since *The Sea, the Sea*. In *Jackson's Dilemma*, he found a precipitous drop in the number of word types Murdoch used, the frequency at which she employed previously unused words, and her range of vocabulary. Remarkably, though, the narrative structure and grammar of Murdoch's books remained essentially unchanged over her writing life, a result that confirms the findings of previous speech studies on individuals with Alzheimer's: even as the linguistic content of patients becomes nonsensical, they continue to produce grammatically well-formed sentences.

In light of these findings, one could argue that even her unintelligible statement to Bayley—"Susten poujin drom love poujin? Poujin susten?"—retains a grammatical structure—enough to entice one to add punctuation, hunt for a code, and discover sound-alike words to substitute for the indecipherable ones.

Still, to insist that the lines *must* make logical sense is to deny the harsh truth of dementia: the disease progressively destroys the very self that used to be capable of love and its expression. It eats its way into your brain, into the frontal and temporal lobes where (in a healthy brain) language is logically interpreted and reproduced. It feasts on Wernicke's area, where meaning is associated with speech sounds and the written shapes of words, gorges itself on Broca's area, where words are systematically deployed in the grammar of a particular language to produce meaning. As the disease waxes, so you wane; as it burgeons, so you contract. Its answer to Murdoch's question "When are we going?" is "We have already left. It is only a matter of time before we arrive."

Ten months after being diagnosed with early onset dementia, I retired from my position as the associate director of the University of Utah's Gender Studies Program. It was August 2011. I had not planned to retire for at least two more years. However, the memory problems persuaded me to leave on my own accord rather than risk a future day when a nervous colleague would pull me aside to discuss some serious gaffe or strange behavior with which I had unknowingly embarrassed myself or the program.

Making serious mistakes was something I feared every day. One of my significant responsibilities during my last two years at Gender Studies had been to compose formal documents about every conceivable area of administration. While our program already had policies for our own administrative and curricular processes, the relevant accreditation body for our program had in recent years started to require the documentation of all policies and procedures according to specific criteria. Since I was the go-to person in our program for policy arcana, I led the effort to bring our program into compliance. I would write the drafts for the various policies with their legalistic definitions and mandates and exclusions, and an ad hoc faculty committee would review and approve them. This work, spread over my last two years, gave me incontrovertible proof of how much my memory had deteriorated.

In order to produce these documents, I had to cross-reference multiple existing university policies. This way of working had been my stock in trade when I wrote research papers for my PhD, corporate memos, and presentations throughout my adult life. I have always enjoyed putting together a logical, well-flowing piece, no matter what the topic. In this new project, though, I found myself haplessly, maplessly lost in a dark wood of legalese.

A new working method soon arose from the gyre of perplexity in which I was trapped: when my task spawned a question, I wrote it down on a worksheet in longhand before switching to the reference screen, so the query would not slip my mind once I got there. The corollary also held: once I found the answer, I jotted it down before returning to my draft. (This tedious method still serves me well as I write this book.) The most stressful aspect of the process was the epochs, eras, eons it ate away in slow motion. For the first time in my life I had to delegate some of my other responsibilities to already overworked colleagues in order to meet our deadlines. While I did manage to deliver the policies on time and well-enough written that my colleagues approved them with only minor changes, my ego was in shreds.

Neurological tests confirmed my experience of loss. While my scores showed that I was still functioning on a relatively high level when it came to vocabulary and verbal comprehension, my working memory left much to be desired. However, during the recursive process of writing, unconscionable amounts of backstage time enabled me to work around the memory lapses and mindboggling confusions, so that even my colleagues did not suspect the efforts that underlay my drafts. Brain research affirms the phenomenon that dementia "is known to disrupt the brain's semantic system, but this can happen subtly before anyone has the remotest suspicion of intellectual decline." During Iris Murdoch's almost twenty-year mental deterioration between her prime with *The Sea, the Sea* and her nadir with *Jackson's Dilemma*, she sometimes "experienced an intense and unfamiliar feeling of writer's block." I can only speculate that her blocks, like mine, were early signs of dementia.

Since our families were very close, my childhood friend Jacoba and I did eventually get together once or twice during school holidays in our standard six year. Though our worlds were growing apart, we still had much to talk about. We also argued: Whose Latin teacher was the best—her Juffrou Holtzhausen or my Juffrou van der Düssen? Who had read the most books in school so far? Whose hostel had the best food? Though I put up as vehement an argument on my own behalf as I could, I inwardly suspected that she was the winner on all counts. My parents came to the same conclusion, after apparently arguing similar issues with her parents, though undoubtedly in the polite, indirect way of adult friends. Consequently I transferred to her school, the Afrikaans Hoër Meisieskool, or Affies as it was affectionately known, for standard seven. Unlike Hoërskool Rustenburg, it was a girls-only school. That it was for whites only as well went without saying.

At Meisies Hoër, Jacoba and I were roommates, sharing with a third girl named Sannie. Everything was as Jacoba had described: the food was more palatable, and served by black waiters wearing the white safari suits and elbow-high gloves that we colonials then deemed necessary; and, humiliatingly, Juffrou Holtzhausen was so far superior to Juffrou van der Düssen that I failed my first Latin test and did not catch up to Jacoba, who was at the top of the class, until the end of the quarter.

School had become far more competitive. By then, though, I had internalized my parents' hubris and expectations about my good brain. Besides, I really liked finding out new things. I even liked the learning by heart that was a cornerstone of South African education: I developed a study method of pleating a piece of lined paper torn from a notebook into four strips, like a fan. That would give me, front and back, eight columns for notes. Grouping the columns into adjacent pairs, I would write a question, term, or portion of a formula on the left and the answer or definition on the right. By folding the paper so that either the left or the right column of a pair faced upwards, I could quiz myself during spare moments. When I felt stressed the night before an exam, I would test myself under the covers with a flashlight after the lights out bell had sounded, rehearsing algebraic formulas, the anatomical names for the bones, or the many tenses of the six irregular Latin verbs, familiar mantras that calmed me down.

After the results of the Matric exam—government-administered tests to qualify for university entrance—were out, my science teacher confessed that she had been on pins and needles about whether I would come through in fulfilling her sevenfold dream for me. In the end I managed to carry the ultimate prize home to my parents: in the nationally administered exams, I was one of only two students in our province who received distinctions in seven subjects, though only six were required for completing high school. My name and picture appeared in the papers, and *Die Transvaler* even published a photo of my father, introduced by the line "This is what the father of a seven-distinction matriculant looks like!"

On the social side, too, things were looking up. With Jacoba, my other roommate, Sannie, and new friends, I was hardly ever

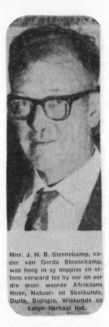

Mnr. J. H. B. Steenekamp, va-
der van Gerda Steenekamp,
was hoog in sy noppies en ef-
fens verward toe hy oor en oor
die mooi woorde Afrikaans
Hoër, Natuur- en Skeikunde,
Duits, Biologie, Wiskunde en
Latyn herhaal het.

Translation of the Transvaler's caption: "Mr. J. H. B. Steenekamp, father of Gerda
Steenekamp, was as pleased as Punch and somewhat tousled and dazed as he
repeated over and over the beautiful words, Afrikaans, English, Natural Science,
German, Biology, Mathematics, and Latin."

homesick. However, my new world of overachievers created other
issues. Math class, in particular, was very stressful. Juffrou Weiss
was an excellent teacher, but came with a strong German accent
and an unquenchable intent of implanting a character-molding
Teutonic discipline into our unruly Afrikaans souls. In between
striking us with her ruler, she practiced a form of shaming that
somehow also encapsulated faint praise. Reading our test scores
from the bottom up, she would pause for effect before uttering one
of her stock statements. "En die *ghres* is *deughr*," or "And the rest
passed."

Once in Juffrou Weiss's class—in the middle of a quadratic root
extraction—I suddenly felt overwhelmed with fatigue. To summon
my energy, I relaxed and unfocused my eyes. Instantly everything

in the room shrank into miniature. At the blackboard, Juffrou Weiss had become the size of my brother Klasie, her gesturing hands pointing to an equation so miniscule I would need binoculars to make it out. The sound in the room was dialed far down, too, like the way my father played his transistor when everyone but him went off to bed. I felt far away and untouchable. However, fearing Juffrou Weiss's ruler, I forced myself back into the present.

Back at the dormitory that night, I tried to replicate what I'd done in class. It worked instantly. The moment I *let my eyes hang loose*, as I came to think of it, *Ecce!*—there was Jacoba's bed, shrunken to the size of the slatted wooden platforms in the showers that kept us from slipping. On top lay Jacoba, as small as the doll that I got the Christmas after my father started teaching and which I secretly wished had been a microscope instead. The hostel was very quiet, except for the housemother shouting at the kitchen staff below. The sounds from my own private puppet theatre were as muffled as the sound in the Bioscope after you had slipped out to the toilet and, on returning, had to wait outside the doors for a loud part in the movie before the usher would let you in again. All I had to do when I wanted everything to become real again was to shake my head and let my eyes just look without thinking about them. Knowing I could make this happen whenever I wanted to made me feel invulnerable, as if enveloped in the full armor of God, even though by then I had embraced my father's atheism.

My dear, I am now going away for some time. I hope you will be well.

Though I don't choose to go to the loose-eye place any longer, "going away" is something that happens to me without warning. I might be in the middle of slicing an avocado when making dinner with Peter; meeting my friends for a cup of coffee; going downstairs to do the laundry (and instead arranging my jewelry by function, metal type, and color in ice cube trays recommended by *Redbook* for the purpose); walking to the front door to answer my grandson's knock (a big-eyed Hennie-Boshoff lookalike with a penchant for launching himself at my thighs so powerfully that my swooping up of his four-year-old body to my chest momentarily becomes the only grammar I can summon for love).

I do not want to *go away.*

Like Iris Murdoch and John Bayley, Peter and I met on a university campus. Like them, we hope to demonstrate that love can thrive in the "uncompromising familiarity" brought about by dementia. There, though, the similarity ends.

Peter and I fell in love at the University of Pretoria in a physics lecture hall, surrounded by two hundred other first-year students, when I was seventeen and Peter nineteen. Since that day, my love for him has anchored me to the wondrous reality of right here, right now. In the months and years that followed, the connection each of us felt in that first moment evolved into a—so far—forty-nine-year relationship, the last forty-five of which played amid the long haul love of marriage. *Going away* was far from my mind, or rather, together Peter and I were already away, borne aloft by the "holiness of the heart's affections."

Redemption has been—is—everywhere, every*when*, as close at hand as the unknown girl we spot out the car window picking up a maple leaf the size of a breakfast plate, as algorithmic as the yellow-gold fall carpet in our yard that we rake into ad hoc nests into which our grandchildren, Kanye and Aliya and Dante, plunge headlong like our children, Marissa and Newton, did in their time, Peter and I in ours, our forebears in theirs, and generations to come will do until the sun becomes a black dwarf and there are no trees to reconsider their leaves, conclude that their verdancy is the price of routing all nutrients to the trunks and roots so they may survive the winter, revoke the photosynthesizing privileges of the foliage (thereby unmasking the golden, orange, and yellow hues of carotenoid pigments hidden all summer by the shocking green of chlorophyll), dispatch a chemical Dear John letter that reads "Go away!" to every leaf, each of which stoically replies with a bumpy line of scissor cells that snips the leaf from the stem until it hangs on by a few threads of xylem so fine that the next breeze launches the golden glider upward on a small, looping whirlwind, which, like a lover on the rebound, soon casts it to the ground.

Where are you going, Gertjie?
  I'm going to play in the sand.

Chapter Four

This Is Your Brain on the Fritz

FAMILY LEGEND HAS IT that on a winter day when it was pouring with rain in Cape Town, my parents sent me into our neighborhood café with the task of buying a loaf of bread. "One loaf of brown bread, please," I was reported to have said. From the shop door Pappa beamed his pride over the cocoon in his arms that was my baby sister Lana, and Mamma formed the words with her lips as when we had practiced them at home. She gestured by her pointing umbrella that I should stretch my arm toward the counter to hand over the money. Exchanging a conspiratorial smile with my parents, the café *tannie* handed me my purchase and the change. As I toddled toward my parents, shedding coins but keeping a determined grip on the still warm, uncut, and unwrapped loaf against my tummy, Pappa announced to the draggle of customers, in the informative tones of a *National Geographic* voiceover, that I would only turn two in nine weeks' time.

Given the nature of legend, it is of course possible that my parents inadvertently misremembered the downpour as winter rain rather than a summer shower, which would have made the event nine weeks *after* my second birthday, or maybe it hadn't been raining at all, but my hair was still wet and seaweed-smelling after a day on the beach, or maybe it was my father only who took me on an excursion while my mother had stayed at home with the new baby. Whatever the eyewitness circumstances, the narrative drive of this family fable is clearly my parents' desire to make known for posterity what they perceived as their first child's extraordinary cleverness.

This and other similar stories, more familiar from their frequent retellings than my actual memories of the experiences themselves, formed the kernel of my "self" during my formative years. As I grew up, I mercifully got over the notion that a strong intellect in my case—or in others', exceptional beauty, or athletic prowess, or musical ability—should constitute the core of any respectable identity. For who or what would you be if accident or injury, moth or rust, should destroy that God-given gift? What in you would be left to declare, "I am"?

However, early childhood impressions, particularly those laid down before the acquisition of language, are—as Freud rightly tells us—impossible to erase. Our "mature" conscious mind may rationalize them away, but our unconscious clings to them like Freud's archetypal mothers to their penis envy. Accordingly, when I received the news that microvascular disease was clogging my brain and gumming up my memory, my first impulse was to use that old standby, my supposedly superior brain—or what was now left of it—to find out what was going on inside my skull. I plunged into a project to find out as much as I could about the human brain.

Note to self: Remember that the poet Virgil who guided Dante through the nine circles of hell did not thereby gain heaven for himself.

Note to readers: If your desire is fixed to follow me, see what is the fate of our cause: All the gods on whom this empire was stayed have gone forth, leaving neither shrine nor altar; the city you aid is in flames. Let us rush into the battle's midst, and die!

PS from Virgil: The only hope of the vanquished is not to hope.

I began my brain project with a refresher on what I had learned in high school biology. In hindsight, "refresher" was a hubristic understatement—my memory, which feels so clear when recalling buying a loaf of bread sixty-five years ago, needed serious jogging to remember the p's and q's of the brain, from pineal gland to quadrigemina. And then there was the whole new alphabet of neuroscience, a branch of brain studies that was only just coming into existence during my high school years in the 1960s. Since science stands or falls by the details, bear with me as I share the know-how that helped me understand my unraveling mind.

The spinal cord, along with the brain, makes up the central nervous system of humans. It partners with the brain to send information around the body as electrical signals. It tells the body what the brain wants and the brain what the body is feeling. In evolutionary terms, we can think of the spinal cord as a proto-brain—it first developed in worms. As more complex organisms evolved, the spinal cord got longer and thicker, eventually needing protection in the form of the spinal column, a tunnel made of vertebrae. All vertebrate animals have spinal cords, from jawless fish to birds and mammals. As animal complexity increased, more nervous system components were needed to send information around larger and more specialized bodies. The resulting new brainware was packed on top of the spinal cord, forming increasingly complex brains. By the time the subspecies *Homo sapiens sapiens* emerged, our brain had grown to almost forty times the weight of the spinal cord, that is, almost three pounds to the spinal cord's one ounce.

The modern human brain consists of three major structures,

which, in the order they evolved, are the brain stem, the cerebellum, and the cerebrum. To imagine how this complex organ came about through additions to the spinal cord, let's mimic the evolutionary steps in modeling clay: First, roll a chunk of red clay between your palms into a rope for the spinal column. Next, make a green knob and stick it on top of the spinal column for the brain stem. An orange wad of clay, shaped to look like a peach, becomes the cerebellum, sticking out at right angles from the brain stem. Finally, shape a large dollop of yellow clay into a mushroom-style umbrella big enough to top the brain stem and cerebellum like a helmet. This is the cerebrum. Last, let's make the newest part of the cerebrum, a thin layer of cells known as the neocortex. Pinch off a plum-sized piece of purple clay and roll it out round and very thin, as you would for a pie crust, until it is almost twice as big as the top surface of the yellow cerebellum-mushroom. Now fit it over the cerebellum, crinkling it up to fit like a shower cap.

Voilà! This is your brain. Sort of.

Now let's take an earth-to-moon step from kindergarten to anatomy 101.

The oldest structure in the human brain, the brain stem, first appeared in our vertebrate ancestors 450 million years BCE. It is located between the cerebellum and the larynx, right behind where we swallow—think of it as the extension of the nerves in your spinal cord into your brain. Given its evolutionary origins, the brain stem is also known as the reptilian brain. Carl Sagan wasn't kidding when he said, "Deep inside the skull of every one of us there is something like a brain of a crocodile." But let's not dis our "crocodile": it forms the link between the spinal cord (our worm brain), the cerebellum (our mammalian brain), and the cerebrum (our *Homo sapiens sapiens* brain). The reptilian brain controls the heart, lungs, and other vital organs. It enables our quick, involuntary reaction to immediate danger and contributes to the control of breathing, sleeping, and circulation. The second oldest brain structure, the cerebellum or mammalian brain, encapsulates the brain stem. (Remember our yellow mushroom umbrella?) First evolved in mammals 200 million years BCE, roughly in parallel with the dinosaurs, the cerebellum coordinates movement, balance, and motor learning. For example, it combines sensory input from the inner ear and muscles to provide accurate control of one's position and movement. The physical slowing associated with depression illustrates how deficits in the cerebellum result in malfunctions we can observe in people's movements.

The newest part of the human brain is the cerebrum or cerebral cortex, which first appeared 2.5 million years BCE when the genus *Homo* evolved. The cerebral cortex (*cortex* is the Latin word for "cap"—ah, our purple shower cap!) is associated with higher brain functions such as complex thought, perception, and action. The neocortex is the outermost layer of the cerebrum, and it's what doctors see when they crack open someone's skull to perform surgery or autopsy. Only found in mammals, the neocortex consists of a six-layered structure of neurons, or brain cells, that occupies the bulk of the cerebrum. It varies in thickness from two to four millimeters, but instead of a single sheet, the neocortex folds over on itself, again and again, forming wrinkles. Its surface area is much larger than the surface of the skull, which enables the brain to pack in millions of additional neurons while retaining a head volume that fits the size of the human body. For now, at least, we have not evolved into creatures of science fiction, with huge dome-like heads and withered bodies. Instead—courtesy of the cortex's wrinkles—we grow from bobble-headed babies to adults capable of supporting and controlling our heads, even as our *Homo sapiens sapiens* brain enables intellectual functioning on a level never before achieved.

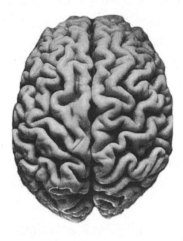

The highly wrinkled neocortex

The more recently a particular mammal species evolved, the more wrinkled its brain appears. In us latecomers, then, our voluminous neocortex has many fissures, grooves, and rounded prominences that bud on the hemisphere surfaces like cauliflower florets.

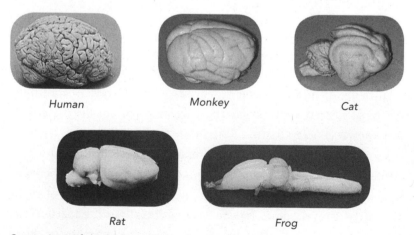

Comparison of the brain surfaces of various species. Note that the frog has no cerebral cortex at all.

The cortex consists of neurons and supporting cells known as glia. A neuron is an excitable cell that processes and transmits information through electrical and chemical signals. A typical neuron consists of a cell body, dendrites, and an axon. Dendrites are thin structures that arise from the cell body, often extending for hundreds of micrometers and branching multiple times, giving rise to a complex dendritic tree. Their job is to receive electrical messages from the axons of neurons. An axon is a long threadlike extension of the cell body that conducts impulses away from the cell. In humans, it can extend as far as one meter.

Structure of a Typical Neuron

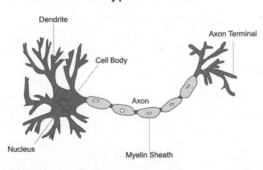

In a living brain, cortical neurons appear gray. Accordingly, clusters of gray neurons on the surface of or inside the cortex are known as gray matter. The brain tissue underneath the cortex looks white, since it mainly consists of axons protected with a white myelin sheath. Clusters of this type of neuron are therefore known as white matter. Clusters of gray matter, consisting of axons that are not myelinated, appear deep within the white matter. The lesions at the root of my dementia are (so far) located in the white matter of my frontal lobe.

The ability to pack more brain matter into the available space in the skull has allowed primates and especially humans to evolve new functional areas of the neocortex, for example, enhanced cognitive skills such as working memory, speech, and language. Working memory is the system that actively holds information in the mind for tasks such as reasoning and comprehension. To underwrite all these functions, the working memory must actively manipulate information rather than merely store it. Why am I telling you all this? This is where dementia comes into play. My own deficits in working memory are the bane of my life, causing my daily failure at tasks as simple as making a phone call.

[Typical progression of a Gerda phone call: (1) Find the phone number (I no longer remember any phone numbers, except now and then my own); is it in my electronic or paper address book? (2) If electronic, open email to search contacts. (3) Forget why email is open, start catching up with unanswered messages. (4) Eventually remember original intention (sometimes). (5) Retrieve number, go to the phone, hear the message beep. (6) Retrieve messages, return urgent calls. (7) Start cleaning the counter where the phone is plugged in. (8) Damn! Who was I going to call again?]

Damage to gray and white matter can cause profound impairment. One root cause of various kinds of brain damage is reduced oxygen flow to the entire brain or a particular area. Any extended oxygen deprivation, such as that caused by trauma, intoxication, stroke, oxygen deficiency, or carbon monoxide poisoning, can be debilitating, even if the person survives the damage. Deprived of oxygen, neurons will be unable to undergo cell division to produce new neurons to replace the damaged ones. In vascular dementia, the oxygen deficiency results because of the blocking of microscopic blood vessels.

Until the 1990s, one of the commandments of neuroscience went "Thou shalt not grow new neurons once thou art born." That changed with the discovery of neurogenesis, or the ability of adult human brains to produce brand new cells. According to our current understanding, each of us grows millions of new neurons during our lifetime, "even as we are elderly and dying of cancer." In order to understand the limits of neurogenesis, however, one has to know most of our daily dose of new neurons do not live very long. To become part of the working brain, a new neuron needs not only support from neighboring glial cells and nutrients from blood, but also, and more importantly, connections with other neurons. Without these connections, neurons wither and die.

During puberty, millions of new neurons arrive in our brains and new connections are formed. Their growth is triggered by sex hormones, and the job of the new arrivals is to prepare the individual for the adult world. The explosion of new neuron growth occurs in the frontal lobe, whose main function is supervising the rear brain. In other words, the neurons that proliferate in the frontal lobe during puberty have the job of developing the so-called executive function, or our capacity to "make social judgments, weigh alternatives, plan for the future, and hold our behavior in check."

On a biological level, the acquisition of neurons involves molecular rearrangements that enable the formation of miles of new neuronal connections. When we exit puberty, our brains will never again form new connections at the rate and to the extent they do while we are teenagers. Our transition to adulthood is heavily governed by the knowledge and skills the prepubescent child has already stored up and connected to related areas of control. If the prepubescent child has missed important peak phases of development—like obtaining language skills, forming social bonds, or acquiring basic social skills—the frontal lobes would face an almost impossible task in rectifying those deficiencies. As adults we can only fully develop our executive function by building on connections we made in childhood and during adolescence. By the age of twenty-five, it's pretty well set.

New research confirms what a lot of parents know intuitively: the teenage brain functions very differently from that of a mature adult. The prefrontal cortex—the very part of the brain in which the executive function, which includes impulse control—is, in itself, in a massive state of flux. (From a neurological perspective, trying teenagers as adults in our legal system makes little sense.)

The implication for adults in all this is this daunting fact: damage to the nervous system in adulthood is irreversible for most practical purposes. Our brains just can't restructure brain matter as quickly or widely as they used to. But all may not yet be lost: research suggests that the most active area of adult neurogenesis is the hippocampus, an area in the medial temporal lobe that distinguishes new events, places, and stimuli from previously experienced ones and appropriately indexes and stores the new ones. The hippocampus is an active area for neurogenesis in adults. Some scientists have proposed that those thousands of new cells produced in the hippocampus each day could be put to marvelous use in restoring the rapidly fading capabilities in my and others' executive functions, but research has not yet shown how, or even if, they can indeed do so. In a radio interview, Michael Gazzaniga, one of the founders of contemporary neuroscience, recently stated that the idea of brain plasticity might have been "oversold."

Dementia Field Notes

6-30-2013

Since our neighbor Bob's stroke during the summer of 2011, his dementia has been getting steadily worse via a series of little strokes, some so small Diane doesn't notice—but his MRI sees

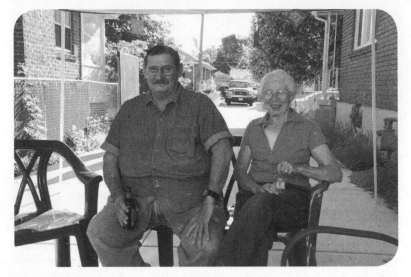

Bob and Diane Bond, my across-the-street neighbors. Peter took the photo during a friends-and-neighbors summer party at our house on July 27, 2009, two years before Bob suffered the stroke that triggered his dementia.

everything. Last week he had a "crazy" episode. While I was outside at the mailbox, he frantically waved me over. He said he was very mad at "her," pointing to Diane, who was peeking out the front door. By then, Diane said, Bob had already been shouting abuse at her for over an hour. He was furious because he thought the paper had not been delivered. She had already finished reading it and had put it in the recycling bin. Even after she fetched the paper, he was not appeased. He told her to call the newspaper office to complain. I suggested that Diane go inside to ostensibly call the paper, but instead call the doctor.

With Diane back inside, Bob calmed down a little bit. He let me hug him. I could feel him relax against my body. I got him to sit down so he could show me where Mary's dog had bitten him a few days earlier. He pulled up his pants legs and pointed out each bandage. Then he remembered being mad, and told the story again. The only thing I understood was this remarkable sentence: "I would prefer that that woman should die." He kept shouting his curse, so I walked him to our house to show Peter his dog bite. Diane returned with a dose of his "mood medicine," which the doctor had told her to double up. Bob refused it. Under our combined cajoling, he reluctantly swallowed it—and slept through most of the night and the next day.

———

Despite my father's ambition and his and my mother's work ethic, they "farmed out," as Afrikaans has it, during the late 1960s. By the time I started high school in 1961, my father, Boshoff, was already in a salaried job away from home, leaving my mother, Susanna, to maintain the farm by herself between weekends. The seventies, though, heralded better times. By the time my parents put the farm on the real estate market, my mother and my two youngest siblings were the only ones living permanently on the farm. While all of us later appertained back to the farm as an edenic time in the Steenekamp family life, it was the natural beauty and the togetherness of our whole family that we missed most. The camaraderie, though, hearkened to a much earlier time, before both my father and I left the farm in 1961 to attend the same high school, he as a math teacher and I as a student. Our joint move did not result in father-daughter togetherness: I was still in the school hostel, my father's commute between town and farm took two and a half hours every day, and our paths never crossed. After my father moved on to an engineering job, I changed schools, and my older siblings started high school, the logistics of coming together as a family became even harder. After five years of disruption and anxiety, we were all happy to put the physical farm behind us. The farm as metaphor is a different matter—divorced from its material signified, it lives large in our memories as "home."

After selling the farm, my father made his way up the career ladder in a whirling series of job changes. For almost a decade after he got his first job as an engineer rather than a teacher, my mother and the younger children followed him from one small town to the next. At last in 1973 he found employment worthy of his engineering education and drive: he was offered a job as a refrigeration engineer with the South African Bureau of Standards. The family—the household now reduced to my parents and two youngest siblings—reassembled in a nice house near my father's work in Pretoria.

The rest of us had ventured into the world to each discover our own "Steenekamp," or "Fortress of Stone." By the late seventies, Lana and I were each living in our own houses, married and pregnant with our first children. Klasie had completed his military service in the Angolan border war (all the while managing to sidestep the army haircut by hiding his locks under a cap or helmet for two years). Carel had submitted to the haircut but circumvented the border by becoming a warden in Pretoria Central Prison, South Africa's "factory of death" for political transgressors. Our youngest siblings were in high school, Hennie-Boshoff going on fifteen, and Tertia thirteen.

While my parents' family life was certainly much more settled than before, time had brought its own new challenges. By the time I graduated from university in 1969, my mother started to suffer from a series of maladies—pain, itching, depression—that her doctors dismissed as "psychosomatic." In those days, even more than today, that was just a polite way of saying it was all in her head. It was almost a relief when about four years into her misery, she was diagnosed with Hodgkin's disease and started undergoing cancer treatments.

Such, then, was the situation on February 23, 1977, Lana's twenty-sixth birthday, when my mother was awakened in the early morning hours by the knock of two policemen at the door. They gave her the news that my father, who was due back that day from a business trip, had died of a heart attack during his flight home. She was to accompany the officers to the morgue to identify him. When

Klasie showed up while the messengers were still there, they told him in a whispered aside that he had better accompany our mother to the morgue. If you die on a plane, they said, the air in your body is pressurized. When you are taken off the plane, you swell like a *vetkoek*, or ball-shaped cake made out of bread dough, when it is dropped in hot oil. Klasie, who had seen his share of horrors during his stint in the army, offered to spare my mother that ordeal. She refused. "Pa's body is part of what makes him Pa," she said. "I lived with that body for almost thirty years." Recognizing a nonnegotiable situation when he saw one, her oldest son drove her to the morgue. She never regretted her decision.

If anyone else showed care toward my mother during those first weeks of her widowhood, it wasn't me. I lived in a town an hour away and was eight months pregnant when I stood over my father's grave with the rest of my family. Marissa was born three weeks after my father's funeral. She would have been his first grandchild. As I examined my daughter while we were still in the hospital, it got through to me. My father was dead. He would never see her. She would never know her Oupa Boshoff. And yet, there he was in her ancient newborn face: his puzzled frown, his spluttering outrage, his benign contemplation of the marvelous world.

After Peter and I had taken Marissa back home to the nursery we had prepared, complete with farm scene curtains and a print of a farmyard with a red cow (a style I would later come to know as American primitive), I vacillated between repressed grief and besottedness with my homemade miracle. For weeks I disappeared into a cocoon of new-mother solipsism. My brothers were each beset by his own struggle to find his way in the adult world. Lana, though five months pregnant, was the one who came to the rescue when Tertia called in the middle of the night to say my mother had fainted in the bathroom and knocked her head on the basin's edge and was bleeding. When my mother was too sunken in depression and the

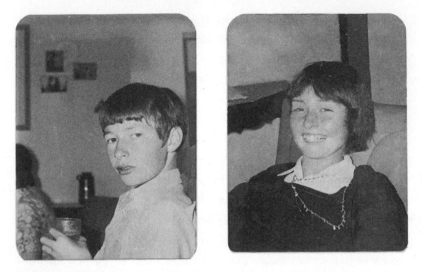

Boshoff, 14, and Tertia, 12. Christmas 1976. Our father died two months later.

aftermath of radiation and chemotherapy to fulfill a mother's role at all, Lana was the one who took Boshoff shopping for clothes.

Somehow everyone got through the hard years that followed. Lana, who lived near my mother in Pretoria and besides, at no matter how large a remove, has a "big heart, / wide as a watermelon," continued to be the primary person taking care of her. Once I had a better handle on parenting, I kicked in on a smaller scale, cluttering my mother's house with baby paraphernalia from eight to five while Peter was at work, or having her over in our town, Kempton Park, for week-long sleepovers, during which we did yoga together while Marissa napped. By the time Lana and I each had a second child, my mother's cancer finally went into remission. My brothers, too, moved on, going to school and/or finding jobs, marrying, and discovering their own niches. Mine, it appeared, was my fascination with my children's unfolding into their own selves. I turned it into a profession, albeit an unpaid one.

Never before had the brain diverted me as much as the two

organs, "fresh from God," inside my babies' skulls. Since Peter was doing well in his climb up his career ladder, I became a full-time mother and observer of child development. I read everything about cognitive, affective, and moral development I could lay my hands on: Jean Piaget's systematic study of cognitive development, with his own children as subjects; Maria Montessori's method of enabling a child to learn independently in a prepared environment; Lawrence Kohlberg's use of Piaget's storytelling techniques to study the moral development of children; and Dr. Spock's assurances that a parent's instinct often trumps that of a doctor and that routine is a good thing as long as you don't become rigid, and his sneaky Freudian insights about the development of the ego.

Mostly, though, I learned from my own children and their playmates. During the day, if I had time, or at night if I didn't, I jotted down the highlights of my children's days like Jane Goodall documenting her chimps. I have kept my data for the seven-year stretch from 1979 to 1985, recorded in 3½-by-4-inch "housewife's diaries" that Northpark Pharmacy—my supplier of plasters (Band-Aids), baby Tylenol, and asthma medications—gave away at the start of each year. Here is a flavor of my WUI (writing-under-the-influence) scholarship:

01-28-1979. [Marissa 1 year 9 months old. Refers to herself as Zaza.] Marissa wants something from the shops.

Mamma: "Pick-and-Pay is closed."

Marissa: "Zaza daddy new car ride. Buy key. Unlock Pick-and-Pay."

08-10-1981. [Newton 1 year 9 months old. Since their births, Peter had spoken English to our children and I Afrikaans. Accordingly, they followed suit from their first words onward.] Newton learns the [Afrikaans] words "kas," "bed," and "stoel." That night while Marissa and I were showing off his new vocabulary to Daddy, Peter does the quiz as directed:

Peter: "What is this?," pointing to each object in turn.

Newton responds [in English], "cupboard," "bed," and "chair."

Like my parents and their story about little Gerdatjie at the bread counter, I now have aren't-they-precious legends of my own. Are mine "better" because they are documented?

Though I'm glad I have my notebooks, what matters about those years, are, of course, not the data, but rather the love writ large in my long-term memory: a daddy who saw to the children's needs to "play rough," who set up pranks, made up bedtime stories about Jo the Schmo and Willie the Fink, and who acquired the first home computer available in South Africa, an Apple I that used a voice recorder as a memory source and on which almost three-year-old Marissa played Frogger. I remember the oumas and aunts and cousins at whose houses they had their first sleepovers and who became their playmates for a day or sleepover buddies for a weekend or a week; a kitchen with worktable and a cupboard of art supplies, where they could play art or math or science any time of the day; shelves brimming with books in almost every room of the house; a pirate's chest overflowing with Lego treasures; a garden with dewdrops on cobwebs, earthworms, leaves patterned with veins, all overseen at night by "the new Moon / With the old Moon in her arms."

Doña Quixote: Parenting gives you a second chance at being a child.

Dementia Field Notes

11-15-2013

Diane had eye surgery. Back home she was supposed to put in antibiotic drops twice a day. She couldn't manage it, so she phoned me. I helped her with it morning and evening for the rest of the week. When she sat on a kitchen chair tilting her head, Bob was very interested in what was going on—he stood behind Diane's chair so close that the side of his body touched mine. While Diane was holding still, he petted as much of her head and shoulders as he could reach, while murmuring unintelligible phrases. His body language and facial expression were loving. Diane wryly remarked that he thought she was his mother.

———————————

The Neolithic Ensisheim skull, found in Alsace, France, and dated approximately ten thousand years old, bears the mark of two trepanations performed years apart. A trepanation is the oldest surgical procedure for which there is archaeological evidence. A healer or spiritual leader would drill or scrape a hole into the human skull to treat diseases such as migraines or epileptic seizures. Trepanning was used almost unaltered until the Renaissance, other than that the drills of each period reflected the technological materials of the time, from rock to steel to diamond. Today, the procedure is known as craniotomy. Neurosurgeons sometimes use it to gain access to brain structures for placing monitors and to relieve the pressure in the skull after a brain hemorrhage. Given the precision of modern bone cutting tools, surgeons cut the hole with minimal damage to the circular "trapdoor." The bone is now placed back in the hole as soon as possible after surgery.

The journal *Archeology* reports that, despite the crude tools used on the Ensisheim skull, the hole "toward the front, measuring 2.6 by 2.4 inches, had healed completely. The second hole had only partially healed, probably because of its enormous size (3.7 by 3.6 inches). The long-term healing evident from the bone…[through] post-surgery regrowth…indicates the operations were successful." In addition, single skulls with multiple trepanation holes have been recovered from Peru to Europe to China. Multiple holes in the same skull, each in a different stage of bone regrowth, confirm that Neolithic patients survived successive operations separated by time intervals ranging from months to decades.

Since no form of metallurgy had yet been invented, Neolithic trepanning holes were cut with a sharp-edged flint knife, starting with a circular or rectangular groove. The surgeon then cut and scraped the bone deeper and deeper until the dura mater, or tough fibrous membrane forming the outer envelope of the brain, was penetrated. The bone removed from the skull was too shattered for the healer to close the opening with it after the procedure. Given that these surgeries were performed without anesthesia or antiseptics and with what today seem like very primitive tools, our forebears' achievement of neurosurgery with a more than 50 percent survival rate is nothing short of remarkable.

How had the man from Ensisheim borne the pain of two trepanations? One explanation is twentieth-century neuroscientists' finding that the bones of the skull and brain tissue lack pain-sensitive nerve fibers. However, certain areas of the scalp, muscles of the head, and blood vessels along the surface of the brain do have pain sensors. Accordingly, as if to concede something to the seeming horror of ancient trepanation, today's craniotomy patient receives at least a local anesthetic before the opening of the scalp, "a prick...like a bee sting." Hospital websites disclose that during the opening of the scalp there will be "a tugging sensation as the skin is cut." The *British Journal of Neurosurgery* reports that the "significant noise and vibrations" of craniotomy drills lead to sensorineural hearing loss. Amazingly, though, patients withstand the surgery tolerably well, even if most of them do need narcotics afterward for up to four weeks to manage their pain, and after that, over-the-counter painkillers and anti-inflammatories for months, sometimes years.

Still, both our ancestors' forbearance of trepanation procedures and modern craniotomy patients is testament to the mind's capability to override some of the most painful sensations generated by our bodies. In the nineteenth century, Sir Charles Lyell formulated the concept in a passage about the evolutionary growth of the minds of animals and man throughout Earth's history:

It may be said that, so far from having a *materialistic* tendency, the supposed introduction into the earth at successive geological periods of life—sensation, instinct, the intelligence of the higher mammalia bordering on reason, and lastly, the improvable reason of Man himself—presents us with a picture of the ever-increasing dominion of *mind over matter.* [My emphasis.]

The relation between mind and matter is today the central concern of the discipline we know as neuroscience, the study of mind. This field has been developing for just over fifty years. At the start of that decade "there was no unifying theory of brain-behavior relationships. In fact, before the 1960s, few neuropsychology practitioners existed."

In 1983, the day came when Hennie-Boshoff and Tertia were both done with Matric, the country-wide government-administered university entrance exam; he was going to medical school, and she was embarking on a career in HR. My mother, Susanna, was fifty-nine years old. She had been a widow for six years, and now her children were grown. She was free. She sold the house, stored what was worth keeping, and took to the road with only those possessions she needed for everyday use. She was yearning for something more exotic than just another "Steenekamp."

Susanna journeyed southward to the birthplace of white South Africa, the Cape of Good Hope. She traveled south at a leisurely pace, stopping along the route wherever she had friends and acquaintances. After reconnecting with relatives and friends in Cape Town, the city where she had lived before our family's move to the farm, she wended her way northeast to Stellenbosch, where she had gone to university and met my father, then dropped south toward the ocean. Following the Garden Route toward the Knysna Wilderness, she scouted out the wayfarer destinations dotting the edge of the continent: the town of Hermanus, where a whale crier bellows out sightings of southern rights mating or calving in the bay; the rocky headland at Cape Agulhas that constitutes Africa's southernmost tip and where visitors cannot resist the attempt to identify the precise ridge of ocean eddies that connect the left-lobe Atlantic to the right-lobe Indian Ocean. She slept over in rural Bredasdorp, which spills down the Preekstoel Hill amid undulating fields of wheat; she lingered in the harbor town of Mosselbaai, where our Middle Stone Age forebears sheltered in caves in the sea-facing cliffs, from where they harvested the ocean bounty, including shellfish brimming with the omega-3 fatty acids that would fuel the development of our large modern brains. At some point, she came to a stop in a picturesque town named for George III, the Mad King of England during the time of Waterloo, a former woodcutters' settlement that nestled in a fertile valley a *hanetreetjie*, or cock's stride, from the coast, a xanadu surrounded by the Outeniqua Mountains, indigenous forests, fast-flowing rivers, lush farmlands, and exquisite *fynbos*, a vegetation type so rare that it occurs only in a hundred-by-two-hundred-kilometer-wide coastal belt that constitutes the Cape Floral Kingdom, the most richly diverse of Earth's six plant kingdoms.

It took only a few days' looking around before Susanna knew she had found her personal "Parke [with] goodly meadows, springs, rivers, red and fallow Deere [gravid with] Fawnes." She bought a house, had her furniture trucked from the Transvaal, and moved in.

The brain's four major prominences are known as lobes. Each lobe is named for the bone of the skull that overlies it. Accordingly these gyri are known as the frontal, parietal, occipital, and temporal lobes. The back three, that is, the parietal, occipital, and temporal lobes, are involved with the input of information into the brain, whereas the frontal lobe is responsible for the output of all information resulting in planned, voluntary actions. According to my MRI report, my detected lesions are (so far) all in the frontal lobe.

The input role of the temporal lobe is primarily centered on hearing. Much of what is known about its functions comes from studying people who have had damage of some kind in this area. In both the right and left hemispheres, the temporal lobe has a small area about the size of a Kennedy half-dollar that is responsible for hearing and is known as the auditory cortex. The temporal lobe is also involved in perception and memory.

Injury to the temporal lobe by disease, trauma, or, most often, stroke can produce a language disorder known as Wernicke's aphasia, a condition characterized by an inability to understand what someone is saying and an inability to read. Injury to the right lobe can result in an inability to recognize and appreciate music and other sounds.

The input role of the occipital lobe is above all associated with seeing. When the occipital lobe isn't functioning as it should, a patient experiences disorders of perception, such as impaired color vision or the inability to recognize objects. Extensive injuries result in blindness. Injury to the right occipital lobe results in an inability to see in the left visual field, and vice versa for the left lobe.

The input role of the parietal lobe is associated with touch and is responsible for perceiving, analyzing, and assembling sensory information from the body. The parietal lobe is the site where visual, auditory, and haptic, or touch-based, information combine to make sense of the world. The left parietal lobe is the area where letters come together to form words and where words are put together in thoughts. The right lobe enables understanding of the spatial nature of the world, including the ability to recognize faces and shapes, be aware of body states and deficiencies, and know directions.

Injury to the parietal lobe can lower the ability to recognize touch sensation from the opposite side of the body. Injury to the right lobe could also result in not being able to recognize familiar objects by touch. Injury to the left lobe could result in not knowing the meaning of words and the inability to do arithmetic calculations.

For the moment, as with the other input lobes, my doctors blame my losses in parietal lobe functions on the output failures in my frontal lobe rather than injury to this input lobe itself.

Learning so much detail about how my daily deficits relate to the material brain cast my dementia in a different light: the dispassionate glare of the scientific method. I had a dysfunctional memory because groups of cells in my brain had died. It was not "my fault" that I had become less reliable and did not pull my weight in the daily underpinnings of running a household. I could see the cause of my failures as white spots on an MRI. Simultaneously, I marveled at the huge, dark blob that showed how much of my neocortex was not yet affected—the blob still included presumably intact cell structures for appreciating new knowledge and the delight it brings—a delight that lasts as a happy feeling, even after the facts have slipped away.

In George in 1983, my mother was settling into her new home. Her real estate agent recommended a young man as a lodger. Neighbors suggested a woman who could clean twice a week and a *jong*—Afrikaans for "young man," the equivalent of the dismissive use of "boy" for black men of all ages—who was looking for a gardening job. With the help, Susanna soon had her new place pulled together: the mahogany table from the farm with its six *riempies* chairs* reigned in the dining area; the dark wood of the Welsh cabinet showed off her Royal Doulton rose-pattern china from the creamy center to the old-gold rim of each petaled edge; the built-in shelves spilled over with her books and art materials. On the table a curiosity cabinet of found objects—a piece of driftwood from a Cape Town beach, an ostrich egg shell, a handful of peacock feathers—awaited transformation into one of her trademark floral arrangements. But first things first: it was spring outside and the yet unexplored environs of the garden and neighborhood beckoned.

On a Thursday morning, when the "garden boy" came, the Old Madam, who was provided for until the end of her life, and the middle-aged *jong*, who was grateful for the job he had found on his afternoon off from the carwash, worked together in a strange harmony: they tackled the overgrown shrubs, the tangled straw of last season's cut flowers, the pebble-strewn area that would become a lawn. Susanna showed him what to toss and what to keep, and even heaped garden debris on the wheelbarrow herself.

When the man left in midafternoon, Susanna returned to the inside cool of her living room and rested in the decadent comfort of her dusty-pink rocking chair. She dozed off right away. A knock at the door startled her out of her nap. A man stood there, cap in hand, asking for coffee and bread. This was not unusual, especially in the *platteland*, or rural parts. The high spiked walls and

---

* Chairs with seats made out of rawhide strips woven in an open lattice. My mother gave me one of the six chairs when we left for America, and subsequently one to each of my siblings.

electrified fences of the well-to-do suburbs had not yet reached George. Susanna told the man to wait and turned toward the kitchen to fill the kettle and cut two inch-thick slices from yesterday's loaf, but before she had even made it across the living room, a lightning storm exploded in her brain. The colors were glorious, winking neon red love-me-love-me-nots, Veronicas firing blue bottle-rockets into the night, Namaqualand daisies dispersing the rings of Jupiter with yellow joy.

A few kilometers away in his office in the business district, Susanna's lodger, too, was experiencing a light storm in his brain: initially unformed flashes of white and gray behind his eyes were turning into the zigzags of battlements like those edging Cape Town Castle. He knew what it was; he had less than an hour before one of his regular migraines would pin him to the toilet bowl for hours of relentless vomiting. He told his manager he had to leave and drove home.

At the house he parked his car and hurried inside. The door was open, and a trail of blood led him to where my mother lay unconscious on the floor. He took her to the hospital, vomiting out the car window along the way. He would spend the next few hours in a bathroom by the emergency room entrance while someone put "Mrs. Steenekamp" in a cubicle, a team of nurses and doctors swarmed around her, and someone called her daughter—the number my mother had given him in case of an emergency was Lana's.

Some of us siblings dropped our lives and carpooled or flew across the seven hundred miles to George. I was not among them—and not because I was too busy. With three of my siblings already on their way, I decided to save my trip. Accordingly, my story of what the others found when they got there is not an eyewitness account, but it may capture the main threads as effectively as any alternative family legend.

At the hospital, everyone was relieved to hear our mother had not been raped. When my siblings surrounded Susanna's bed, her face lit up, though she could not really see them. Her vision was at best a blur of movement against a screen of static, but the doctor said it would improve. After being somewhat reassured by our mother's usual stoicism as well as clear signs that she recognized everyone, the siblings went to Susanna's house to sleep, but not before attempting to erase the map of our mother's ordeal by scouring the pool of blood from the living room carpet where she had fallen. They scrubbed the wine-dark trail from the dining area where she had dragged herself, and mopped the puddles and smears from the kitchen tiles where she had eventually collapsed after the man—who had hungered for much more than coffee and bread— had sliced his axe through her scalp, cleaved her skull, slipped the blade through her dura mater, and slid it into the gray and white matter of her occipital lobe. He fled with her radio, leaving her for dead.

When Susanna was discharged from the hospital a week later, I flew down from Pretoria with her then four grandchildren in tow: my own two as well as Lana's pigeon pair, two girls and two boys between the ages of three and six. What could I have been thinking? But my gut feeling turned out to have been right: what my mother needed most was to be surrounded by the happy chaos of young life. When the grandchildren's arguments about who got dibs on the second pink reclining chair got loud and physical, Susanna abandoned her own chair and went to her bedroom to nap. At mealtimes she reveled in the higgledy-piggledy, and when it got loud and physical she intervened with moral tales intended to instruct and delight. In the mornings when she felt her best, she solicited the children to draw or paint with her. When the children tired of that, we would set out for a drive crowned by a nature walk to collect treasures: seed pods split and curled like the horns of an impala, rocks that glowed like jewels when you licked them, flowers and bones, feathers and bits of glass that had "suffer[ed] a sea-change / Into something rich and strange."

Before the children and I left for home, I extracted my mother's promise that she would not open the door to anyone unless she had first verified their identity. She said she wouldn't, but I suspect that she continued her life just about exactly as before, locking when she remembered, going out into her garden whenever it called to her, venturing on long solitary walks to collect the flotsam she found so irresistible.

On the juridical front, the matter was concluded with the characteristic efficiency with which the apartheid government meted out justice to blacks: in just over a year, the attacker had been caught, found guilty, given eighteen years in prison. Because he admitted his guilt in court, he was spared from the gallows. It was he who chopped the "Old Missus" with an axe, he confessed. He was sorry. It was the *dagga*, the *witblits*, the devil.*

After the attacker had been sentenced, learning of his fate had no observable effect on Susanna. When I pressed her on how she felt—by phone from our home in Johannesburg—she said she hardly ever thought of him or the attack. She mentioned that it felt strange to think that someone was in prison because of what he did to *her.* She was far more interested in talking about her improving eyesight, her drawing and painting, her reading and meditation.

Despite her outward cheer, there were subtle signs that Susanna Before and Susanna After were different: for example, she never made the floral festoon that she said she was about to start arranging after the children and I returned home.

---

* *Dagga* is the name of a South African species of marijuana, *witblits* a raw spirit, colorless, and with a powerful punch.

*   *   *

Soon after Peter and I had emigrated and my mother's move to George, she asked me to "teach her how to write." We concocted a plan whereby she would write stories about her childhood and I would edit them and provide comments. So started a precious communication between colleagues. (I had not yet published anything at the time.) In her stories, my mother referred to herself by her childhood name, Susanna. (As an adult she had become Susan.) I loved the way her given name bridged our separate generations.

As a new immigrant, I was at the time very conscious about names—in the United States mine had become a big stumbling block. It seemed to me that, unlike people who live in multilingual countries, Americans would not even try to pronounce my name. (When I eventually made close friends, I saw that this was not universally true.) Not hearing people other than Peter say my name made me feel invisible. It affected my sense of self. On an associated level, I understood something of how the farm laborers and domestic workers of my childhood must have felt when they were given a "white" name to replace their unpronounceable original. My namelessness also made me think about old people who had nobody still alive who called them by their name. I was surprised about how much the loss of my name affected my sense of self.

With these thoughts in my mind, I suggested that I address my mother as Susanna in our "writing class." She was delighted, so we did it. From that time onward, I frequently thought of my mother as Susanna, even though I addressed her as Ma face to face. After her brain injury in George and later, as her dementia became obvious, I remembered how much she loved being Susanna during our intense long-distance closeness. Since my mother was already confused about who I was, I squashed my impulse to give her back her name. For this reason, as I write about her now, I refer to her as Susanna, except where the nature of our relationship must be stated for clarity. It is my homage to all the selves that Susanna accumulated in her life beyond being somebody's something: a friend, gardener, scholar, philosopher, artist, and writer, to name a few.

A dozen years after Susanna's brain injury she had, via a number of other houses or retirement centers, made her way back to Pretoria and was living, with Lana's help, in her own house in a retirement community. Other than ongoing problems with her vision, she showed no obvious signs of brain damage, though she did from time to time exhibit odd behaviors that we chalked up to her lifelong eccentricity and the fact that she was getting older. At the age of seventy, she was still well enough to travel. Accordingly, for the summer of 1995, she set out to visit us in Salt Lake City.

When I arrived at the airport on the date scheduled for Susanna's arrival, there was no sign of her among the passengers at the baggage carousel. I had her paged, coaching the announcer on the exact pronunciation of her name—people have trouble with Steenekamp. After numerous pagings, she still failed to materialize. Growing more uneasy by the minute, I enquired at the airline's desk. They were not allowed to give me any information, not even whether she had boarded the flight. After I explained her age and the distance she had traveled, the woman at the desk told me Susanna had not boarded, though she had been listed as a passenger on the flight. Sick with worry, I tried to call Lana from a pay phone, but had no luck making an international call. I went home, connected with Lana, and learned that my mother had left as planned. By then, the next plane that came in from her connection city was due. I hurried back to the airport. This time, I spotted the beacon of her all-white hair among the travelers descending the escalator in the arrivals area.

My joyous welcome lasted only a few seconds before my relief turned into anger. As if she were a teenager who had broken her curfew, I started interrogating her: "Where have you been?"

In a tone suggesting that my obvious annoyance was totally inexplicable, Susanna said nonchalantly that she had been looking around the stores and missed the flight.

"Why didn't you call?"

"I don't know how to. I knew you would come for me if I caught the next flight."

Trouble soon reappeared. After we arrived home, Susanna seemed literally unmoored. While out on walks, which she insisted she could do on her own, she often lost track of her whereabouts and had to knock on neighbors' doors for directions. Another time, she urgently needed a bathroom while still blocks away from home. She knocked on a door to ask if she could use the occupants' bathroom. Fortunately, in a city chockfull of serving or returned Mormon missionaries, Susanna's accented modulation of English did not have the door-in-your-face effect it might have had in other large American cities. Her natural charm and defenseless look—more marked as she got older—probably helped, too.

The good outcomes of her wanderings confirmed Susanna's belief that the world was a good place. Even after her axe attack, she had clung to this. Should I have wanted to stop her, it is not likely she would have listened. Her father had walked the mile to and from his vegetable gardens every day when he was already in his late nineties and totally blind. Who was I to fight those genes? At home, her insatiable drive to make art—as if she were racing the clock before a deadline—took over our living room, where she worked at the single-bed-sized study desk I had acquired for my exclusive use. By the end of her visit, she had completed enough paintings and sketches to bestow one on each member of our family and every friend who dropped by. My painting, a twenty-by-twenty-four-inch landscape featuring a quiver tree in the foreground, still enlivens a wall in my study. I thrill to the presence of a tree so evocative of our family's visits to my Kalahari-based grandparents.

In between bouts of sketching and painting, Susanna wrote a journal that would turn into a memoir of her life as a child. By the time she had to go home, she had filled a legal-sized notebook with her memories and thoughts. Once she had typed up the novella-length product on my computer, she shared it with me. It now circulates in our family as bound copies of *Die Mooiste Plekke: 'n Meditasie (The Most Beautiful Places: A Meditation)*. As she writes in the book, it owes its inception to an abstract pencil sketch she had made by scribbling lines across the page and then accenting shapes that stimulated her imagination. "The story of my life can be read from beginning to end in the forms my hand involuntarily created," she writes. "Somewhere in the middle of the composition the picture story starts to materialize."

While I had heard my mother's stories of her past throughout my life and read the handful she wrote down soon after our emigration with the idea that I would "teach her to write," I had never experienced anything like the outpouring of thoughts and feelings that radiated from every page. With—to me—startling awareness of story structure, she organizes her narrative by using her pencil sketch as if it had been a plotting tool: each of the four selves that had materialized in the sketch gets its own name. Switching between the first and third persons, my mother tells each self's story and accounts for the transformation from each one to the next. First comes Susanna, the child who grew up on the banks of the Grootrivier, or Orange River. Her family lived at Kafferswart, a settlement north of the river. "On school days, my father used to awaken me and Pieter early in the morning and gave us bread and coffee," she writes:

> In winter it was still dusk-dark when we walked to the boat, where my uncle and cousins were waiting. Uncle Aalwyn rowed us across. On the other side of the river the school bus took

us a further nine miles to the school at Karos. In 1934, flood
waters swept along everything in its path, including the little
garden with corn and beans Susanna had planted. Their Jant-
wak house on the riverbank is also gone. The floodwaters had
hurtled everything away, including the boat. For the rest of the
quarter there was no school. But there were new islands of sand
next to the red dune skirting the northern bank to explore.

Susanna's halcyon days of endless play ended when she left for
boarding school at the age of eight. When she was nine she heard
her father telling the story of her birth. It ended when "the woman
caught Susanna between Truia's legs just as she was about to drop
on the floor." For the first time, it occurred to Susanna that she
"had emerged from the shameful, private place between her mother's legs" in the same way lambs drop from a ewe. For many years
she would feel uncomfortable when her mother addressed her by
her pet name, "my little lamb."

After internalizing the "fall" of the circumstances of her arrival
on Earth, Susanna is no longer called Susanna in the manuscript.
She becomes Nonsanna, or Nun-sanna, represented by a slight
female figure—a nun—kneeling in the center of the sketch. She
fears that she cannot hold to the rigid strictures of Afrikaner
farming society: children should be seen and not heard; idleness
is the devil's ear pillow; white girls don't climb trees, go barefoot,
read novels on Sundays, wash their hair when they're having their
period. They don't go to university.

After high school, Nonsanna works as a lawyer's assistant in
Upington, a town seventy miles from the farm. After a year of sav-
ing money for university, she sees that she will never reach her goal
with her meager income. She obtains a loan at the bank, which
her father has to cosign. She gets a ride home with a farmer, who
takes her as far as Abeam, a family settlement that was still about

twenty miles from home. There she waits for someone—anyone—traveling deeper into the Kalahari. She spends the night and the next day helping the farm woman with her family's laundry and washing and ironing, all the while scanning the horizon for signs of the dust plume that would signal the approach of a vehicle.

When at last the dust cloud rises, it comes from the wrong direction, the direction where from her father's farm lay. It is slow-moving, too slow to be someone on horseback. A donkey cart? She saunters toward it, slowing her pace to counteract the feathery hope still fluttering in her rib cage. The closer the cart comes, the greater grows her disbelief. But—yes—it is true: the people on the seat are her teenage brothers, Pieter and Kerneels.

Since there had been no rain that year, they had to fetch water for the animals from more and more distant sources every week. Early that morning they had set out, not yet sure which of two alternate sources they would tap. When they got to the fork in the road that led in the two different directions, they let the donkeys decide where to go. The animals chose the road to Abeam.

Back home, Nonsanna does not have to point out the resonances between her rescue and the Bible story of Balaam and the talking ass—it is on everyone's lips. Surely that is a good omen. Their family lives by the Bible. When she broaches the loan with her father, however, his focus is on the verse in the Bible that warns against usury, or the taking of interest. He refuses to sign.

During the bone-shaking ride back to town with a fortuitously passing neighbor, Nonsanna realizes she is no longer Nonsanna. Her name now is Sanna Capital I, or "Sanna must out!" Back in Upington, she approaches her employer who, though an observant Jew, has no truck with the Bible's interference in educational progress. He cosigns the loan. At the start of the academic year, Sanna I travels to the University of Stellenbosch wearing a pair of homemade leather shoes.

As Sanna I studies to become a social worker, she is transformed into Hosanna, represented in the pencil sketch by the head of a woman who emerges beyond a bird burdened by a stone on its head. Loosed by a wind from behind, strands of hair escape from her combs and stream out in front of her face. Underneath the woman's chin is an identical second chin, beside her neck an identical second neck, suggesting a second person moving forward in synchrony next to the first.

"Angels and people sing songs of praise," Susanna wrote in her legal pad. "Who are angels and who are people? Hosanna! Hosanna! After that comes the open end. An open end, because history continues after we arrive at an anticipated end point."

We celebrated my mother's seventy-first birthday just before she left Salt Lake City when the leaves started to turn in August. The end point to which she was heading was her final five months of relative independence: in February 1996, she would be struck with the catastrophic breakdown of her mental faculties that signaled the obvious onset of her dementia.

Doña Quixote: Eternal, and eternal I endure. / All hope abandon, ye who enter here.

Located in front of the brain just behind the forehead, the brain's frontal lobe is above all associated with sending output related to the planning, initiating, and controlling of purposeful actions to other brain areas as well as the body. It is through connections to the brain stem and spinal cord that it controls voluntary movement. Through complex connections to all parts within the brain, the frontal lobes are also involved in controlling attention and concentration, abstract and complex thinking, decision making, mental flexibility, higher judgment and reasoning, and emotional responses. The frontal lobe is where my lesions are the most apparent.

When the frontal lobe fails to do its job, weakness and even total paralysis can result on the side of the body opposite to the injured lobe. Injury often results in distractibility, difficulty concentrating, inflexible thinking, simplistic or "concrete" thinking, the inability to plan or think ahead, poor judgment, and inappropriate emotional behavior.

I am afraid many of these symptoms are evident in my lack of concentration and bumbling behavior. I used to be known as a very focused person. For example, when I was working on my PhD, I did not have a spare room at home to set aside for my research. Instead, I studied at the largest surface we had, namely the kitchen table. During those years, Newton was in elementary school and, later, junior high. Being highly sociable, he had friends over almost every day, and I managed to concentrate despite the roughhousing and noise that frequently enveloped the kitchen space. Now, though, I seem to have an intense form of attention deficit that prevents me from being able to make a cup of coffee, go to the bathroom to brush my teeth, or get dressed without many memory blanks, detours due to distractions along the way, and lapses in focus during conversations.

I fare similarly badly when it comes to "do[ing] arithmetic calculations," and "knowing the meaning of words." In my 2010 neuropsychological evaluation, my first, my neuropsychologist, Dr. Janiece Pompa, wrote that though "Dr. Saunders…had a degree in math,…[she] could not remember the elements of problems long enough to solve them." In my 2012 evaluation, Dr. Pompa reported that "Dr. Saunders's generally good test performance is very discrepant from the serious memory and speech difficulties she describes in her life, some of which were observed during the interview and testing."

As far as "controlling all purposeful actions" goes, in my 2012 evaluation Dr. Pompa noted a complaint about which I had told her, the odd response of my body while I am making decisions: "While walking, she inadvertently wrapped her legs around each other and almost tripped herself." Here is an example of how I perceive this kind of bumbling while walking toward the back door, considering whether I want to go out the garage (as I first intended) or, in a change of mind, fetch the hammer that belongs in the garage and is lying on the kitchen counter three yards away in order to put that in its proper place. My lower limbs seem to follow the vacillation of my thought, "wrapping...around each other" as they try to steer me in both directions at once. Whatever the actual pathways are in my brain when this kind of clumsiness happens, the malfunction causes me to lose my balance or, particularly when my arms are involved, knock items off tables or countertops as my hands shoot out without waiting for my conscious volition to direct them.

Injury to the left frontal lobe in Broca's area—a region responsible for producing language output such as speaking and writing—can result in a language disorder known as Broca's aphasia, where the individual has difficulty communicating with others. Such individuals may not be able to speak or communicate at all or may, even with a great deal of effort, be able to say only a few simple words. While I have been troubled by gaps in my speech when the topic about which I was holding forth just disappears from my head in mid-monologue, and I experience long moments during which I cannot find a word or a circumscription for what I want to say—as I note in multiple entries of my Dementia Field Notes—I oddly am still able to write, albeit much more slowly.

While my MRI does not show any damage to my temporal lobe, I do experience a disruption between the auditory input my temporal lobe presumably receives without too much trouble (my hearing is good when I wear my hearing aid) and the output from my frontal lobe, where the auditory information is processed. On February 7, 2012, I recorded a Dementia Field Notes entry that serves as an example: "I just heard the term 'clinical trial' on the radio. I could not figure out what it meant. What came into my mind was a forensic trial, something like CSI investigators testifying in court. (I Googled CSI—it means Criminal Scene Investigation.) My head took far longer than is useful in conversation or writing to work itself around to the recollection that a clinical trial is 'a blind study of medications.'"

In similar fashion, while my occipital lobe presumably has not suffered any damage, I sometimes have problems with seeing. I attribute this to the inability of my frontal lobe to process the information my eyes send it. In an apparent confirmation of this mechanism, Dr. Pompa reported in 2010 that my test scores "suggest excellent retrieval of information from visual memory, while [my] recognition of visual information was below average." I guess, therefore, "mis-lookings" are the fault of my frontal lobe.

Dementia Field Notes

07-25-2013

When I put away my salad bowl after lunch, it appeared oval rather than round. I turned it the other way and it still looked oval. It made me feel disconnected from myself—as if it were not me looking at the bowl. I took a nap, then checked the bowl again. It was round.

———

What most puzzles me about my incipient dementia, though, is that even as the failings I describe above slow me down and stress me out in my daily tasks, my head still works well enough for me to write. A clue to this discrepancy may lie in Dr. Pompa's explanation of a similar discrepancy between my performance on everyday tasks and achieving above average scores on neuropsychological tests. "It may be that her superior intellectual ability allows her to perform well on tasks in the office setting," she wrote in 2012, "which are structured and controlled by the examiner, but that she has considerably more difficulty when required to attend to, remember, and organize the details of her everyday life."

Dr. Pompa's breakdown of my scores became more plausible to me during a 2013 vacation with my family in South Africa: while I was noticeably scattered in looking after myself and my possessions—on two occasions I left behind indispensable medication, left my purse in a mall bathroom (the lady who had used the stall after me found it and she and the attendant chased after me to return it), and regularly knocked over my wine or coffee—I was nevertheless able to communicate almost nonstop in mostly intelligible language. The reason? Because of my memory difficulties and clumsiness, my brothers and sisters, Peter, my children and their spouses, and even my grandchildren took over all responsibilities associated with keeping thirty people fed and happy when we—my siblings and their families—gathered at the seaside. At home, I have no choice but to spend a big chunk of mental energy doing my share in our household; in South Africa, I could devote this to keeping my head together.

Doña Quixote proposes a toast to the family:

The family—weavers, reachers, winders
and connivers, pumpers, runners, air
and bubble riders...
...soothers, flagellators—all
brothers, sisters, all there is.
Name something else.

*   *   *

Peter's and my plans to emigrate had taken root long before my mother's axe attack. We had considered the possibility from about the time Marissa was born in 1977. Was apartheid South Africa the best place to raise her? Or would it be wise, should we be able to succeed, to emigrate? When Newton was born two and a half years later, these questions intensified: as a boy, he was destined to serve in the interminable war between South Africa and the "communist" insurgents believed to threaten the country not only from its entire northern border, but also from within: the Oliver Tambos, Steve Bikos, Desmond Tutus, and Nelson Mandelas touting the absurd notion of a nonracial society.

When we managed to keep our blinkers on, life in our new house in Parktown North, Johannesburg, was good. Peter had his own one-man computer consulting company that he ran from our repurposed entrance/dining room. Newton was a chubby toddler, Marissa a lanky preschooler, and they played out their days in the beautiful walled garden we had laid out. I was still a "professional" mother, who, by then, had gained Lilliputian fame among friends and acquaintances as a supposed expert on staging what my friends regarded as educational happenings, but were really just play that involved science and art at the same time. Since I played in this way with my own children in any case, it seemed to make sense to sometimes include children of a friend, a neighbor, or acquaintance. After once holding an extravaganza on the solar system and space travel for about six elementary school children, I submitted their work to an art contest then running at the planetarium. I'm proud to say "we" won most of the prizes.

Outside the cocoon of our home and wider circle of friends, things were not so idyllic. An apartheid-fed social turbulence seemed to spiral ever wider into our white lives. Three incidents in particular stand out as triggers that turned the notion of emigration from an abstract possibility into a necessity. The first arose out of the apartheid pass laws. Rose Mnisi, our twice-a-week housecleaner and resident sage, lived in the servants' quarters in our backyard, which consisted of a small, cement-floor bedroom and a toilet/shower cubicle situated across the paved area outside our back door. Rose's daughter Maria, who was nineteen, attended a teacher training college a day-long train ride away. When she visited her mother during vacations, she stayed with Rose, an illegal act: her pass, or government permission to live in a particular area, was not valid in white Johannesburg.

As was customary at the time among self-described enlightened white anti-apartheid suburbanites, Peter and I welcomed Maria and undertook to help Rose watch out for the police, so that Maria would have time to hide under Rose's bed or in our house should they come sniffing around. The event that would disrupt our lives, however, came not in a house call by the authorities, but rather in Maria's not unreasonable desire to experience life outside our walled yard and locked wrought-iron gates. Despite Rose's strict fiat to the contrary, Maria one afternoon ventured outside the gates. Just a block or so from the house, she fell prey to an enterprising policeman who inspected her pass and, upon finding it wanting, promptly confiscated it. His act deprived Maria of her legal identity. She could not even return to the area where she legally lived. The price for getting the pass back, the young man said, was to sleep with him.

When Maria returned home passless, terrified, and crying, Rose's only plan of action was a threat to beat her. When Maria begged me to take her in the car and help her get her pass, Rose agreed that this might possibly be more fruitful. With Rose next to me in the passenger seat and Maria and the children in the back, we drove around the neighborhood looking for the officer. Within minutes Maria spotted him. He appeared young enough to have barely completed high school. Emboldened by my decade-plus age advantage, I got out of the car, searching my mind for an argument suitable to the absurdity of the occasion. Rose, too, got out. Before I could use any of my supposed "White Madam" power, Rose accosted the young man, drenching him in a torrent of Sotho, the vituperative nature of which was unmistakable even to me, who knew only a sprinkling of words.

Rose's verbal abuse and hand gestures apparently invoked me, since after looking at me with what looked like fear, the young man wilted. He produced a handful of passes from an inner pocket and handed them to Rose. After making sure Maria's pass was among them, she confiscated the remaining documents. She would announce them at her church, together with the officer's name so that someone would be sure to tell his mother, a shame that caused the young man to slink away before Rose had worked off all her anger. What remained, she spent on Maria: she was not ever to leave Rose's side and, should Rose have to do an errand outside the gate, she would be locked in their room.

The second disturbing event also involved the police, but the representatives of the law were much less amenable to threats than the pass confiscator had been: they were two white men. I would encounter them one day while I shopped with Marissa and Newton in the strip mall where I shopped for groceries. Since parking was always an issue, I felt lucky to find a spot in the same parking lot but some distance away from my destination beside a restaurant in the same complex. As I scrambled out with the children in tow, I did not take particular note of the vehicle next to which I had parked—that is, until five-year-old Marissa, pointing to the police van, asked, "Why does that man have blood on his face?"

As I took in the situation, my heart went cold. The van was stuffed with black prisoners, apparently on their way to jail. What Marissa had picked out as unusual was that the man at the open but barred window had a streak of not quite dried blood across his face. His injury did not seem too serious, the blood apparently emanating from a small wound over his brow. I registered, however, that he was gasping for breath. A gap the size of a Bible was left open on either side of the van. While on a cool day it might have been adequate for one person, the temperature was unusually high that day, and—even worse—more than a dozen other prisoners had been piled into the van like circus clowns into a Volkswagen. Those whose faces I could see were straining toward the meager source of air, all the while squeezing the man by the gap ever tighter.

I did not know what to do. *Water?* I grabbed my children by their hands and set out for Pick-and-Pay. As I was about to cross the parking lot, I spotted two officers finishing their meal in the shade of the restaurant's overhang. Without considering what confronting two policemen could bring—we were already then feeling that we lived in a police state—I marched the kids toward the officers and accused them of leaving the prisoners in a hot, airless van while they sat down for a meal.

One of them, an Afrikaans speaker, lost no time in berating me for my ingratitude that he and his partner were risking their lives to keep "us whites" from being murdered in our beds. He followed with sarcastic remarks about how he wished that *he* had the time to go shopping with his children. In the meantime, the other officer was squatting down at the level of my children. In the interested tones of a favorite uncle, he asked their names, then scribbled the information in his notebook. Where did they live? What work did their daddy do?

As fast as possible I yanked my kids away and hurried to get them back in the car. Their interrogator, however, followed me. By the time I had found my keys, the man was in front of my car, pointedly copying down my registration number. What he might do with the information I could not even imagine, though scenarios of knocks on the door during the small hours and the arrest of Rose and Maria, or even Peter and me, raced through my head.

The third incident was the most disturbing. A day or so after Peter and I had attended a party at my sister Lana and brother-in-law's house, one of the guests told Buzz that he had been contacted by the security police. Apparently he had made a remark at the party that was unpatriotic and smacked of a threat to the state. Given that both the person approached and Buzz were employed at the uranium enrichment division of the Atomic Energy Board where I myself had worked after graduating from university, it did not seem utterly implausible that the security police had indeed made the call. What seemed utterly incomprehensible, though, was that someone among our *lifelong friends* would have reported him.

Against this background, getting out of South Africa took on an urgency we had not felt before. Shortly after these incidents took place, Peter made a business trip to a client in Salt Lake City, a company then known as Sperry and soon after as Unisys. To Peter—as to the thousands of tourists who vacation here every year—the city seemed magical: snow-capped mountains, friendly, utter absence of crime. Half-seriously, half-jokingly he asked the American team leader whether Sperry had a job for him. The man took his overture at face value. A short while later, the company flew the two of us out to look at suburbs and schools and house prices. I, too, fell in love with the Mormons' gentile Zion. Peter accepted the job. All that remained was obtaining a work visa. A month or two later, we got word that it had been granted. Ignorant as we were about the then already hellish bureaucracy of the American immigration system, we did not realize that the type of visa that had been issued for Peter was nearly impossible to upgrade to the holy grail of a green card. Two years into our move, we turned into illegal immigrants. It would take eight years of intensive personal and legal effort before we could hold our hands to our hearts and pledge allegiance to the flag of the United States of America.

That we were eventually able to become US citizens is an ironical happiness: if it hadn't been for the excellent education Peter had received in South Africa as a privileged white person, he would never have been sought-after in the computer field to the point of his company paying thousands of dollars for emigration lawyers so that they could keep someone with his skill set in their employ.

Peter and I made our decision to emigrate at about the same time that my mother was planning her move from Pretoria to her then yet-to-be-decided-upon destination. When we told Susanna that we were going to live in Salt Lake City, she was happy for us. There was, however, something in her eyes other than the vacant look we often saw after her axe injury: a deep sadness, it seemed, about the vast distance our move, on top of hers, would put between us.

Where are you going, Gertjie?

I'm going to play in the sand.

In my memory, my father still persists as the person who stood for logic and rationality in our family, while my mother personifies imagination and the sagacity of seers and sybils. What my father, by the time of our emigration already dead seven years, would have thought of our leaving the country of our birth, I can only imagine. But I hope that since he left the farm for the city under sociopolitical and environmental circumstances, he would know it was in the best interest of our family. As for my mother—now that I have grownup children with their own children, I am only beginning to fathom the wisdom and generosity with which she managed to see our plans to settle ten thousand miles from the formative valley of the Steenekamp farm.

In George, however, all was not well. While Susanna had recovered physically from her injuries and on the phone she said she was fine, it seemed that her former irrepressible drive to find adventure had dimmed. In "the flow of energy between two biologically alike bodies, one of which has lain in amniotic bliss inside the other, one of which has labored to give birth to the other," I sensed—or did I project?—a preemptive, existential loneliness about the great distance my family's move to America would put between us. But there was another quality of sadness around my mother too, a more ordinary desolation: the grind of daily life without those you love most dearly nearby.

After we had said our final goodbyes—the most wrenching of which took place at the airport on the day of our departure—and after the thirty-hour plane trip during which Marissa's feet had swollen so much she could not get her shoes back on and thus arrived barefoot in America, after our weeks-long stay in a residential hotel in Salt Lake City, and after we had settled in our house on the shores of prehistoric Lake Bonneville, Susanna once more set out from George. Even her relentless drive to turn negatives into positives had not been able to overcome the irrationality of the sociopolitical circumstance of her environment. Summoning "the flow of energy between two biologically alike bodies"—this time herself and her mother—she moved to the Karoo village of Marydale, where her parents had moved after retiring from their Kalahari farm. Her mother, Truia, was in her early eighties, her father, Carel, ninety. Carel was blind, Truia lame.

They used to think she was ouderwets.

Though Carel and Truia adamantly asserted their self-reliance—Carel followed the fence with his fingertips to tend his vegetables, and Truia oversaw from her wheelchair the *hotnot* woman who cleaned and helped with the cooking—Susanna felt that the time had come for her to take care of them.

As soon as she had made all the arrangements to return to the landscape of her childhood, Susanna recruited my brother Carel,

who owned a *bakkie*, a small flatbed truck, to move her possessions the 375 miles due north. So far did the weight of her remaining memory-steeped worldly goods exceed the *bakkie*'s payload,
though, that its bed sank almost to the tarmac at the back, causing
its headlights to beam drunkenly skyward, all the while continuing
to lurch fecklessly into the unseen territory that "danger knows
full well." By contrast, Susanna, who had become accustomed to
not trusting her eyes, followed the timeless beckoning of the North
Star to her kismet, even though from her southern hemisphere vantage point that beacon was obscured by the lobe of the earth's crust
and the bulk of its mantle.

You give your heart to each thing in turn—Ma's little lamb.
After that comes the open end.
Hosanna, Hosanna.

Chapter Five

Of Madness and Love I

Love is the fourth kind of Madness.

PLATO, *PHAEDRUS* (249D)

*What indeed is madness but the orgasm between conscious-
ness and unconsciousness.*

J. F. C. FULLER, *THE BLACK ARTS*

I SAW MY FIRST MAD person when I was almost five years old. We
had just moved from Cape Town to the Transvaal and were living
with my father's parents in the Old House on the farm. We couldn't
have been there more than a day or two when I came face-to-face
with Willeman. Our cousins, who lived within walking distance,
were visiting. Hendrik and I were the oldest of the bunch, and we
ventured out to explore.

Out toward the tobacco barns, the *werf,* or area of swept dirt surrounding a farmhouse, ended in a tall screen of quince trees. To get
around them, we first had to pick a path through a treacherous quilt
of quill-sharp, inch-long, V-shaped thorns that studded the earth
beneath a giant tree called a *pendoring.* The two-pronged thorns
called *dorings* resembled the straight, sharp horns of a gemsbok,
a kind of large antelope. After managing to toe our way around

the nasty spikes unharmed, Hendrik and I raced toward the row of quinces. When we came around the hedge-like lane, I froze, and the image before me would be etched into my soul: a man with red, bulging eyes; hair matted and sticking out like a mane; torso bare from the waist up, except a sash knotted from small-animal skins that was looped around his chest; a mantle of sackcloth, adorned with bits of fur, feathers, leaves, and bones, swung from where the sash crossed over one shoulder. And then there was the smell: a bitter mix of tobacco juice and sweat, overlaid with the tang of rotting animal. He was surrounded by a pack of yelping dogs, which he thwacked from time to time with his stick. The dogs picked up their pace, and so did the madman.

My legs sprang back to life, and I ran. Hendrik, who grabbed my hand as he tore along beside me, bellowed an earsplitting warning: *"Dorings!"* He braked with a dust-raising skid that threw me off balance, and I stumbled to the ground. The madman was catching up with us. He stopped, stared, and laughed, his mouth open so wide that you could see the back of his tongue and the spaces in his gums where he was missing teeth.

This time Hendrik did not stop to take my hand. I tore after him blindly, seeing only the back of his shirt as he swung far to the side of our ouma's front garden to give the advancing front of man and dogs the widest berth possible.

Having gained the garden, we saw that the man had not followed us. As if he had never even noticed us, he had continued to the back door. (I would later learn that he went there for food every day.) We slowed, followed the outer rim of Ouma's plantings, a row of bushes with red flowers. Hendrik showed me a secret hiding place under the low branches, a den, he said, that was handy when your parents were looking for you after you had been naughty. We crawled inside, wincing at the sharp ends of broken branches poking into our sides and backs.

Once our breathing became quiet, I asked Hendrik about the

man. His name was Willeman,* Hendrik said, a moniker I would only later realize was not a real name, but rather the Afrikaans for "Wild Man." He was a *sangoma*, or witchdoctor, Hendrik continued breathlessly. He wore a string around his neck; suspended on the string was a bag containing bones that, Hendrik said, he threw to make black people sick or even make them die.

"Bones?" I asked.

"He gets them from the people he kills," Hendrik ventured, his sky-blue eyes wide. "After he throws his bones, he lets his dogs eat them. He has to kill someone else to fill up his bag again."

The alarm he must have read on my face drew a reassurance from Hendrik. His *muti* did not work on white people, he insisted. Then he told the funny part that he had saved for last: each of Willeman's dogs was called Voertsek, an Afrikaans command used to chase dogs away.

Inside our hiding place, a snake suddenly slithered over Hendrik's foot. My big cousin screamed and ran. I screamed, too, and ran right back into the thornfield. I stepped hard into a *pendoring*. Wailing, I hopped to the back step of the Big House.

Hendrik's mother, Tant Tien, offered to take it out. All I managed in response was a sound that meant "Don't come near me."

When my father came home from the lands, he did not take no for an answer. He told me to sit still, or else someone would have to hold me down. I cried out when the needle would slip into the quick, upon which Pa, undeterred, joked that it was a wonder the jackals out in the veld did not join in.

While I soon forgot the pain of the thorn extraction, one certainty burned onto my brain: Hendrik was wrong; Willeman's dark powers were far stronger than my whiteness.

---

* Hendrik recently told me his name was "Pietman," but Willeman was how I had thought of him for decades.

*   *   *

A characteristic of brain injury, whether caused by disease or trauma, is that it leads to unexpected patterns of skill retention and loss. A 2013 *New Yorker* article by David Owen includes an anecdote illustrating the vagaries of brain injury. Owen writes about "a gifted structural engineer" who can no longer practice his profession because he "lost his ability to remember new things." He nevertheless retains "amazing" math skills and the ability to play chess. If the former engineer momentarily leaves the chess game, he cannot remember whether he was white or black and, upon returning, has to infer his color from where his opponent is seated. Remarkably, he is then able to look at the board and "retrace the game backward and then run it forward," and in this way "he will almost always beat you."

Today it is commonly understood that the particular way in which a mind goes wrong is inextricably related to where the damage is located in the brain. However, this concept had no traction in neuroscience until about two decades ago. The failing to pair up "local changes in tissue content with cognitive and behavioral changes" was due to a cultural blind spot: the reign in the first half of the twentieth century of behaviorism, a theory that human behavior (and the behavior of other animals) can be explained in terms of conditioning, without consideration of thoughts or feelings. Behaviorism entailed the belief that psychological disorders should be treated by changing behavior rather than delving into the human mind.

Under the reign of behaviorism, the brain came to be regarded as a kind of black box, an organ of "*mass action* (the brain as a whole determines its performance) and *equipotentiality* (any part of the brain can carry out a given task, thus no specialization)." Before contemporary neurology could flourish, the vast cultural-conceptual notion that mental and physical processes were, in Stephen Jay Gould's term, "non-overlapping magisteria," or fields of knowledge incapable of casting any light on each other, had to be overcome.

*   *   *

I saw my second mad person during our last year in South Africa, when Newton was a four-year-old in preschool and Marissa a seven-year-old second grader. Like most white parents in the area, Peter and I transported our children to and from school by car. At pickup time, the parents—almost exclusively mothers—would stand around chatting while we waited for the final bell. Our preschool-age children, those who stayed at home or who had been picked up at their private nursery schools along the way, played together under the trees. In a separate group, the nannies who stood in for the mothers who were having their hair done, were delayed at their doctor's offices, or—rarely in those days—holding a job, conducted their own conversations, which were always louder and merrier than those of the white madams. Their own children and grandchildren were forbidden by the pass laws to live with them on their employers' premises. They had to send their offspring to townships or "homelands" to be raised by grandmothers or aunts and attend substandard schools.

One day a white woman whom I had not seen before appeared under the trees. She was accompanied by a black nanny, dressed in a uniform pink from apron to *doek*, who was pushing a white baby in a pram. Although the baby's two caretakers each belonged to a different conversational constituency, they did not join either group. The baby looked very new, so I decided to walk over to congratulate the mother. With a nod at the nanny, I asked the mom, "How old is your baby?"

"What baby?" she responded. She averted her eyes and fixed them on a toddler running a stick backward and forward along the fence.

The nanny wheeled the pram closer so I could peek inside. "He's a boy, ma'am," she said. "He has two weeks."

Without coming any closer, the mom said, "That's not my baby." Though her tone was emphatic, her blank expression did not change. The nanny reached out to pat her employer on the shoulder, and the white woman again settled her gaze on the toddler. Turning to me again, the nanny introduced herself as Regina and explained they were there to pick up the woman's daughter, Addie, then went on to share the baby's eating and sleeping patterns, topping it off with a report of his sister's naughtiness. "When I give him the bottle," Regina began, "Miss Addie, she throw me with crayons. She don't like I have another child on my lap."

The mother injected herself into the conversation again. "That's not my baby," she insisted. "Somebody else's baby. Just looks like him."

Just then the grade ones were let out, and amid the fracas, Regina waved goodbye and so did I. We often chatted after that. The mom never again attempted to speak to me, though I always made a point of greeting her, too. Instead she stared blankly into the playground and jumped when the wind swirled up papers or a bird flitted through her field of vision. I did not ask about her oddness. Regina did not explain—if, indeed, she had an explanation.

As the semester drew to an end, I sought Regina out almost every day. She always rewarded my complaints about all the work related to our packing and leave-taking for America with an "Auwk! Poor madam." From her side, Regina confided about the baby's steady growth and increasing cuteness—"He smile at me and he sister this morning"—and also filled me in on her own children and grandchildren back on the farm. Poppie, her seventeen-year-old, was applying to the Normal College to become a teacher. Joshua, her married son, lost his job at the factory and was at the moment living illegally with her in her room, but—with a glance at her employer—madam did not mind because he hid from the pass police all day and only went out at night.

When the term ended, I was sad to say my goodbyes to Regina. She, too, seemed emotional. She said she wished she could one day come and visit me. I told her we would be honored to have her as our guest, though we both knew such a trip would be virtually unfathomable. As we touched in a handshake, we both teared up. I wiped my cheeks with the back of my hand, she hers with the point of her *doek*. As we parted to each take our own grade one girl by the hand, she glanced at her employer, the baby, and his sister, who was goo-gooing into her brother's face. Regina sought my gaze, held it while imparting her last words: "Sorry, ma'am, I won't see you for a long time. Not until I've raised these ones up."

During the time I got to know the mentally ill woman of whom Regina was taking care, I had no inclination how big a role madness would play in my own family. While my children were babies and toddlers, my mother was ill with Hodgkin's disease, but no one imagined that her biggest health challenge would be the loss of her reason. I was a young mother, immersed in life challenges both intellectual and practical, with no inkling that I myself, together with Peter and our children, would get to know madness from the inside. I now look at my mother's dementia with a more intense personal interest than before my diagnosis.

After Susanna's mental collapse in 1996 and once she had somewhat regained her reason, she actively and bravely grappled with her unnamed deteriorating condition. She, like me, resorted to writing: Once she had been resituated in the old-age home, Susanna began keeping a *dagboek*, or daybook: "I walked throughout the sick time for exercise," she wrote in one entry. "I slept through the afternoon for the lack of inspiration or initiative to do something better." "My illness brought the finality of things, events strongly to the fore. Is that what is crushing me?"

The twenty-seventh and final entry of Susanna's daybook is the only one with a title: "Die Ware Jakob," or "The True Jacob," an Afrikaans expression for "The Real Thing." The entry was intended to replace her many false starts on a memoir she had mentioned she was composing, a putting-to-paper of her "justification" of her life. At the time of the last entry, she had apparently lost all the work she'd done on the computer. While awaiting help to relocate her files, she wrote a longhand "true beginning" of her memoir, which I found in her room after her death. Her writing stops midnarrative. She never again wrote any prose we know of—only her name.

The last entry differs from the previous ones in several respects: Susanna writes on every other line of the ruled page, whereas she did not skip lines before—and on this day she wrote one-quarter of the entire daybook. The writing seems fevered—the spacing and orthographically drawn-out words reminiscent of my own long-ago blue book exams. The content, too, is atypical. This entry alone is devoted entirely to her illness.

When I started reading my mother's daybook, a retroactive dread cramped my heart. How could it be that she suffered so much confusion and unhappiness without me understanding the depth of it? Nevertheless, with an impulse akin to that of John Bayley when he keenly observed his wife's indignities, I continued reading: I wanted to know my mother's dementia in all its awfulness. I did not then realize that a similar fate awaited me. I also did not anticipate that I, like Bayley, would decide it was okay to make my mother's distress public. After I had joined the unenviable club to which my mother belonged, I, like Bayley, convinced myself that shining light into the lonely and scary place of my mother's dementia—and mine—could possibly be of value to other people who live with dementia, whether it's their own or that of someone they love.

Die Ware Jacob

4-28-1997

The illness last year from beginning February to the end of October and everything I associate with it—which proves that it did happen—will not leave me. Whether I deny it or whether I affirm it or whether I just let it be…it drags behind me like a specter, is always with me.…The dreadful anguish and shock when I realized I would have to live in an old age home for the rest of my life left me with a fragile heart. Life would never get better.

The night before the onset of the illness, I was working on a painting, inspired and enthusiastic: it was a natural scene, like heaven might have looked like, with beautiful plants, flowers, birds, insects, a lizard, and a snake.

It was late when I went to bed and during the night I saw a vision of heaven. Now, for the first time, I think it could have been a dream with a remnant carrying over into the next day like the painting I had made—however, initially I was convinced that it was a vision, a hallucination! This insight makes me feel a lot better. A hallucination sounds much sicker than a dream…Nothing will persuade me now that it had not been a dream!

Now with the telling I realize that I cannot remember the chronology well at all: I came back home from the hospital, but I don't know if I stayed at home. I know I was back at the sick bay, because I got into trouble for wetting the floor. I did it to bring down my body temperature. Something I had successfully done at the Little Company of Mary's Hospital, but on a smaller scale. Back in the sick bay I started getting confused. Or had it already happened at my home?

Even though I have been able to return to my house, the heartsoreness is deeply lodged and I connect it to more and more things. I have the horrible feeling that I was not as sick as it is alleged and that I could have been spared all the trauma of moving. I want to know why I could not just as well have been sick and mixed up at home and have recovered here?

I suspect I must have been ill, since I was so totally dependent and submissive that I did everything I was told.

Reflection on Dementia Field Notes of 5-4-2011

Now that your grandson Kanye has abdicated the portable crib, his sleepovers require more adult accommodations. Accordingly, you are on the hunt for a sleeping bag. Not the Disney kind, with fabric slippery enough to slide, child-and-all, from futon to floor. You want a proper sleep sack, commercial-free and stay-put. Tilting at this newfangled windmill, you set out for Ikea. Before leaving, you study your Google map enhanced with Peter's penciled-in notes. You are Doña Quixote preparing for a quest.

You conquer the I-15 on-ramp. Eyes peeled, you watch the exit numbers fly by. Ikea is just a few exits south from Newton and Cheryl's. Next weekend they're bringing the grandkids for a sleepover: one-year-old Aliya all red-cheeked in her head-to-toe onesie in the crib, four-year-old Kanye snuggled on a mattress in whatever you're going to find and buy today, maybe something like the quilt you stitched for Marissa by tracing her body on butcher paper.

Damn, you missed a road sign! You fix your gaze on the road, proceed gingerly. Suddenly you realize that you have forgotten the number you are supposed to be looking out for. You probe the passenger seat for the instructions, bring the paper level with the top of the steering wheel, snag the number, repeat like a mantra. YES! Only three exits to go. *This place has only three exits, sir: Madness, and Death. As for me and my house,* we shall shop. You will never know whether you indeed took the wrong exit or whether it was the road-work detour that deposited you beside a field dotted with horses, sheep, and winter-gray hay bales. The horse that limped away from its more youthful companions and stopped by your car was the perfect Rocinante to your Doña Quixote. Eye to eye, the two of you contemplated the way home.

You remember the winter rescue of a pod of beluga whales trapped near a Chukchi village off the Bering Strait. It was during your family's first New Year as sojourners of the northern hemisphere. Surrounded by twelve-foot-thick ice, three thousand white whales took turns breathing in a few remaining unfrozen pools. The ocean was beyond their reach, receding as the ice advanced.

Many weeks after the villagers had radioed for help, the icebreaker *Moskva* cleared a channel to the ocean. Weak and bewildered, the whales fed in the larger pools the *Moskva* had made. After gaining strength, they started frolicking to what 1820s explorer William Parry had described as "shrill ringing sounds not unlike that of musical glasses played badly." They swam and they ate; they clicked, yelped, chirped, whistled, and trilled. As the Russian daily newspaper *Izvestia* wrote in despair, they did everything but pursue their escape along the newly gouged canal. At last someone recalled that whales react acutely to music. The ship's gramophone was fired up. Russian folk dances, martial fanfares, and classical crescendos poured off the deck. While the patriotic strains left the whales nonplussed, the classical music did the trick. The herd began to follow the ship.

You love this story. However, you feel that those Russian journalists *left everything out. Turgenev wouldn't do that. Checkov wouldn't do that. There are in fact Russian writers you never heard of, as good as anyone, who would not leave out what they have left out.* What was the music that persuaded the whales? Beethoven's soaring architectonic structures? Mozart's witty contrapuntal complexities? Wagner's unresolved Tristan chords?

Einstein now gets on your case: Wagner? His musical personality is indescribably offensive. Beethoven is too personal, almost naked. You left out Bach! Listen, play, love, revere—and keep your trap shut.

Now a character from graduate school, literary critic Harold Bloom, strolls into your field of stagnation. Scratching the suborbital depression between Rocinante's eyes, he remarks, Don Quixote can remain a hero only as long as he retains his crazy will to be himself, as long as he keeps up the war against Freud's reality principle.

If remaining yourself means you must fight reality, you decline. You, Gertruida Magdalena Saunders, must live and die by reason. Fact is, you have no idea how to retrace your path home along the cambered moonscape pockmarked with half-a-dozen "scattered bifrontal lobe nonspecific white matter lesions." And you know that in this reality, no *Moskva* will materialize for you.

So: You call Peter, cry a little bit, and follow his voice home.

———————

Bob has Diane.

My mother had my sisters, Lana and Tertia.

The woman at Marissa's school had Regina.

Willeman had his dogs.

I have Peter.

After having known Peter for more than twice as many years as I did not know him, it feels as if he has been in my life always. But there was a beginning, a moment when "our souls touched, quivering [me] to a new identity."

Against anyone's expectations—my own included—my love of science won me my first chance at romance: during my Matric year, I scored among the top fifty in a countrywide voluntary science test, an achievement that resulted in an invitation to attend a week-long youth science conference in Pretoria.

In a milieu populated by like-minded science enthusiasts in a ratio of ten boys to every girl, I felt different than at my all-girls school. Daring. Among total geeks, my stunted social skills suddenly seemed surprisingly adequate—or so thought a certain boy (I'll call him Malcolm). He was light-years beyond me in social adeptness. He was also a bit older, eighteen to my fifteen, since he had stayed on at his school to do a post-Matric year.

I met Malcolm after a lecture, when our group was invited to examine a poisonous red spider from Namibia. In the ensuing scramble for a close-up view, I found myself next to Malcolm, who proved his social savvy by saying something clever about the red skirt I was wearing. Before the week was over, Malcolm and I had spun an amorous web out of the gossamer encounter—if holding hands and promising to write to each other once the conference was over could qualify as amorous.

During the Christmas vacation, Malcolm visited my family on the farm. He traveled by train to Marikana and spent a well-chaperoned week as a guest in our house, sharing my three brothers' bedroom while I bunked with my two sisters. Despite being constantly surrounded by my siblings, by whose unending jostling for his attention I was alternately annoyed and pleased, we did have some private moments, one of which led to my first kiss.

Malcolm, in turn, invited me to his home so I could be his date at a country club dance. While I had visited the homes of school friends who moved in more elevated social circles than my family, in Malcolm's house I found myself amidst a level of financial comfort so much taken for granted that no ostentation was necessary. The furniture, though in beautiful shape, lent the house an air of having been lived in comfortably for many years—it reeked of solidity and longlastingness and dogs. I had my own bedroom, where I was served morning coffee in bed by a staff member in a happy floral uniform with a frilly cap. Personal privacy seemed to be taken so seriously that the toilet was not only in a separate room from the bathroom, but also had a tiny entrance hall with a door before you got to the actual toilet. (Vacillating between embarrassment and admiration of Malcolm's adaptability, I thought of him having to share our single all-purpose bathroom with the eight of us.) Mealtimes in his house brought another set of new experiences: a table set with an array of silverware at each plate, a full breakfast in the morning, and dinners for which Malcolm and his father dressed in at least a fresh shirt, often a sports jacket too, and pulled out the women's chairs. The three courses, together with wine, all served by a staff member in uniform, were apparently as quotidian as my family's noisy meals, served on our everyday plates and which my mother often conjured from a single fifteen-ounce can of pilchards (sardines). At Malcolm's house, even the dogs had their own matching tea bowls—brought in on the tray with everything else—from which they were served the milky dregs from everyone's cup before the second round was poured.

A benevolent god could not have dreamed up a setting better

suited to my British-historical-romance-cultivated love map than Malcolm and his family. Thanks to the examples of non-affluent heroines handling themselves well at the homes of "quality," I was only a bit nervous in the beginning before settling in and enjoying every minute of what was the closest I would ever come to a weekend on a Jane Austen country estate, complete with a dazzling ball. As for the sartorial aspects of the crowning evening, I wore the Matric dance dress my mother had sewed—and blended right in.

One year after the country club dance with Malcolm, I found myself in an environment as different from that experience as *Clueless* is from *Emma*: I was back in high school, this time as a senior in small-town Iowa, USA. During Matric I had been accepted as an exchange student to the United States in the American Field Service (AFS). Despite looking forward to this adventure for over a year, being in an American high school was strange, made even more so because I had by then been attending the University of Pretoria for a full semester. Nevertheless, I was still younger than most American seniors, sixteen—almost seventeen—when I suspended my university degree in July 1966 and got on a plane (my first flight) for the US of A.

During my one semester at university, I did have something of a social life. No hearts were broken, however, when I set out to live with the Henning family in Breda, Iowa. My American dad, Al Henning, was a five-foot-five-inch-tall large-animal veterinarian. He often took me along on his rounds, where I, conveniently tall, was made to hold up IV bags or hydrating bottles for cows and calves, lift a cow's tail so that Doc could stick his gloved arm into her vulva to inseminate her with semen from a prize bull, and assist in the birth of twin foals that each had to be dragged out with handcuff-like clamps attached to a front leg on one end and affixed to a chain drawn over a pulley at the other. My American mom, Dorothy, was a "homemaker" who had a bachelor's degree in home economics; she is the person I still try to emulate in my efforts to run our household smoothly and economically. Dorothy helped me make South African *koeksisters*, or deep-fried braided pastries dunked in a thick syrup, as a contribution to the "international dinners" in which I and the other exchange students participated. Joyce, my fourteen-year-old American sister—a high school sophomore—helped me navigate school and taught me to ride a horse, and Beth, her twelve-year-old sister, whom I helped with her math and who shared my love for science, completed my host family.

And then there was the America outside the Henning home.

What is there to say about an adventure that opens one's eyes to the wider world in a way no book ever can; that even in conservative rural America, there reigned a spirit of discovery and striving and independent thought that exceeded everything I had experienced in Afrikaner-run Christian National South Africa; that, from a distance, apartheid looked far worse than it did from inside; that once you left the protective bubble of home, all bets were off. Decoding American teendom was much more challenging than the AP physics course I took.

Item: While growing up in South Africa had equipped Ignoramus Abroad with plenty of stereotypes related to race, a combination of her disinterest in sports, attendance at an all-girls school, and lack of access to American teen movies has left her innocent of the jock/cheerleader categories. Ignoramus is astonished to see the frenzy of attention paid to school athletics, which is almost exclusively focused on boys. Girls' sport-related ambitions seem limited to joining the cheerleading team. Those who get in are automatically elevated to the top of the female social hierarchy, which—as she soon figures out—nevertheless forms a distinct second tier to that of the stars on the boys' teams. From these two top ranks comes the homecoming, prom, and other school royalty. The next step down in the hierarchy is occupied by band geeks, and, bringing up the rear, the Pep Club, including Ignoramus, who—before you can shout "Our Boys Are the Best!"—is declared an honorary member and presented with a Pep Club sweater.

Item: Thanks to Carroll High's previous AFS student, a Mediterranean beauty from Greece who was outgoing and vivacious and had a stunning head of glossy black hair that she could toss as well as any cheerleader, the popular girls are inclined to—sometimes— give Ignoramus the benefit of the doubt: she is invited to a slumber party or two, but never the mixed-gender parties about which she knows through the grapevine. When Ignoramus stages the teen party that AFS students customarily hold at their adoptive homes, however, the popular girls come, bringing along the boys. They seem nonplussed by the fact that the Henning parents make their presence at the house known before retreating into the den and that there is no alcohol in the punch or anywhere else. While the music Ignoramus has carefully selected with the help of her sister Joyce goes down better than the punch, without the spike from that beverage it is just not greasing the social gears. Or maybe American kids just don't dance? Or maybe—

Jock, approaching Ignoramus: Would you like to dance?

Ignoramus, getting up: Yes, thanks.

Jock: I'll go see if I can find someone who will dance with you.

Item: Ignoramus is invited to the homecoming dance by a boy from her English class who is not handsome, a sports participant, or an academic high roller. He is, however, a funny, friendly, and caring human being. Neither he nor she broadcasts their date. For a reason she still cannot fathom, Mr. Knott asks her in front of the speech and rhetoric class whether she is going to the dance. Before she recovers her composure, her date volunteers that he is taking her, the look on his face that of a lottery winner. Several popular girls approach her afterwards, murmuring approval.

Item: Ignoramus, to her delight and surprise, is asked to the next dance by a basketball jock, also known for his witty remarks in class. Her date provokes discussion among the popular girls, who speculate (within her hearing) about why he had not made his intentions known to them. They nevertheless give their blessing to the match. The spring prom, though, proves to be a cipher on a different Rosetta stone. The big event is coming closer and closer with no invitation. She invites an American "cousin" from her host family who goes to another school, who responds with such apparent discomfort that she thinks he does not really want to attend. She makes a deal with him that he will be off the hook should a date with someone else materialize. In the meantime, a phone call comes from a boy at her own school, a football player. Her conversations with him until then had been total dead ends, and she foresaw notes pleated into fans, this time likely diagrammed with football plays. She guiltily declines. (When, as an adult, she gets to know Big Guy a bit better, she realizes saying no had been a mistake: he turns out to be a funny and friendly person who became an English teacher and wrote science fiction on the side.) As far as her refusal goes, it doesn't even occur to her that people other than her family would know about the invitation. The next day at school, though—

Popular Girl: I hear that Big Guy is asking you to the prom!

Ignoramus, taken aback: How do you know?

Popular Girl: I told him to ask you. I thought you'd say yes.

Ignoramus: Unfortunately I had to say no. I have actually made other plans.

Popular Girl: Maybe he should ask Curly-haired Cheerleader. Tallest Football Star just broke up with her.

An unanticipated phone call spares Ignoramus and (formerly?) Reluctant Cousin the set-up solution. This time it is Football-Star-She-Really-Likes. She says yes. They have a good time, she thinks, even though she would not allow his hand in her bra. Fatal mistake, apparently. He never calls or talks to her again.

With hindsight and information gained from a Carroll High reunion about twenty years into our life as Americans, I realize that my high school peers had really mostly been good people, as insecure as I was, though they expressed their self-consciousness in a different cultural vocabulary.

It was some comfort that the town's adults loved me—at least as a speaker. In rural Iowa at the time, exchange students were sought-after speakers. Even formerly non-English-speaking students who cringed at the thought of speaking publicly were obligated to their community sponsor—Rotary International was mine—to give at least one speech during the school year. Unaware of the entertainment value of foreign visitors from students to missionaries, at the time I credited my self-perceived maturity for my appeal, but today I believe that, in addition to the fact that I surprised everyone with my "good" English, the real reason was my exoticism as a white person from Africa—which astonished many people—and the fact that my somewhat formal behavior had originated in a culture that, according to Americans, had been outdated since the start of the twentieth century. Whatever the reason, I was invited to and accepted more speaking engagements than any other AFS student before me and won top honors at the Iowa State Speech Contest.

Like the nineteenth-century female orators who traveled from town hall to town hall to spread word of the women's rights movement, I had found my voice.

It was a much more socially confident me who returned to Pretoria in July 1967 to resume my bachelor's degree. Outwardly, I took more care with my hair and was more daring in my dress than before—the minidresses I brought back from the United

States, mostly items I had knitted or sewed myself, were shorter than those generally worn by my South African peers. An obvious change had also taken place in my auditory self-presentation: I had acquired an American accent.

In the hostel and on campus, the students in my year now seemed very young. Other than my roommate, I did not make new friends for almost the whole semester. For most of my day, I was among strangers. A week or two after the start of classes, I walked into the physics auditorium, still without a friend to look for. I stood in the aisle, looking for a place to sit when, above the subdued pre-lecture murmur in the hall, a familiar laugh sounded. In the section of seats beside me, I spotted a guy with dark, curly hair whom I remembered from a class the year before. We had never really spoken, though we might have said hello to each other once or twice. One of the few English speakers in our predominantly Afrikaans university, he used to hang out with a small group of other English speakers. Amid the blur of still-unfamiliar faces, he seemed like an old friend. I climbed the aisle steps to one row above where he was sitting, and, brashly squeezing past a number of students, took a seat behind him.

I was pulling books from my bag when my chemistry textbook slid off my lap and dropped to the floor. I stuck my head under the desktop to retrieve it. A pair of sparkling brown eyes met mine. From the way gravity distorted his upside-down face and turned it pink, I gathered that my carefully applied makeup was probably not my most notable facial feature at that moment. I muttered something about narrow desks, apologized for being clumsy, and profusely thanked my somewhat-acquaintance who was now holding on to my book's other end. He laughed. "Where did you get that American accent?"

Did that mean he remembered me from the year before? Before I could explain my accent, a swell of clapping signaled the arrival of Professor Verleger. We craned out our heads to see him being wheeled in on an office chair by a graduate student, who set the chair into a spin, upon which the professor began dramatically swinging his arms, slowing or speeding up like a ballerina, to illustrate the conservation of angular momentum.

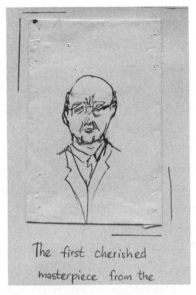

Peter's sketch of Professor Verleger
while attending a physics class, 1968

Nobody was more surprised than I when, after class, my under-the-desktop friend followed me out and introduced himself as Peter Saunders. That day we walked just a short distance across campus together, but a day or two later he met up with me again and, finding that we lived in the same direction, we walked together all the way to my hostel. The apartment block where he lived with his parents, he explained, was just around the corner and across the railway line. Soon enough we found ourselves almost always walking home together. Not that serendipity didn't have a role in this astounding development; we were both enrolled for a BSc degree, and our classes, as well as our three-hour lab sessions on weekday afternoons and math tutorials, followed the exact same schedule. Like most BScs, we had Friday afternoons off so that we could study for the three-hour tests held every Saturday morning. Alone with my books in my room—my alluring roommate had multiple suitors and was frequently out on dates—I worked as hard as I could to avoid thoughts of what Peter might be doing on his weekend. On weekdays, by contrast, I knew exactly where he was: he was with me.

Over the span of weeks, I learned about Peter's family and childhood, and he about mine. He had gone to Boys High, the Pretoria English high school that was socially paired with the English girls high school. His mom was Afrikaans and his father English. Dudley Saunders had worked all his life as a carpenter for the South African Railways, building wooden coaches of the kind that would later supply stunning backdrops for films such as *Murder on the Orient Express*. Raaitjie Saunders, who had always been a housewife, had, from the time Peter started at university, worked as an office administrator at the government lab that, among other things, tested the alcohol content of suspected drunk drivers. Peter's older brother, Cliff, a radio reporter (who would a few years later become a household name in South Africa), was married and his wife, Ria, had just had a baby.

I also learned about a goal on which Peter was very much focused at the time: buying his own car. He already had quite a bit of money squirreled away from his earnings as a magician at children's birthday parties over many years. He had learned to drive long before the legal age of eighteen, using the spacious grounds of the South African presidential estate as his own speedway—for that is where his family had lived until they moved into their flat a year or two earlier. Previously they had shared the house of the groundskeeper during the presidency of Blackie Swart, South Africa's first president after it left the British Commonwealth. The groundskeeper's wife had been his mother's second cousin, and Raaitjie had promised the young woman on her deathbed that she would help raise her two little girls.

Peter and I even knew the names of each other's childhood pets. His constituted a menagerie that included several dogs—one of which he had taught tricks—and also, from the avian class, a crow that pecked his ear in the mornings to wake him up, a house-dwelling chicken or two, a gander that attacked visitors, and a baby ostrich.

At the end of the academic year, Peter and I said goodbye without making any plans to see each other until the next school year. After a short while with my family, I returned to Pretoria to work at the Atomic Energy Board, a condition of my full scholarship. My vacation accommodation was a mattress on the floor in the flat of a friend of a friend. The flat was near a bus stop where I waited every morning before work, a forty-minute drive away. It was also near the university hostels, which meant that it was close to Peter's place. Though I knew he would be in Cape Town, my heart beat faster whenever I spotted a dark, curly head bobbing some distance away on the sidewalk, only to sink into disappointment when the face never was his.

Near the end of the holiday season, though, one of the bobbing heads looked more and more like Peter the closer it came, until it appeared that I was on the mark. He was delighted to see me—the feeling was mutual—and had me point out my flat and give him the number. The next evening he came to visit. We were alone. Before I knew what had happened, we were in the middle of a passionate kiss. When we said goodbye, we knew we would not see each other until

the start of school, which was a week or so away, because I was about
to go home to the farm for a few more days. There was no discussion
about our future relationship.

Though not in quite the way I had imagined, our relationship did take a new turn once school started. One day, with what
seemed like studied nonchalance, Peter invited me to his home
for tea with his parents. I immediately loved them. They were
welcoming, full of fun, curious about everything to do with our
university life, and wonderful talkers, particularly Raaitjie. They
spoke about what was going on around them in the world rather
than offering news-related opinions or abstract philosophies.
Most astonishingly, they were physically demonstrative, frequently touching each other lightly or exchanging looks of pleasure or amusement. In the kitchen, while we were clearing tea
things away, Dudley lightly kissed Raaitjie on the top of her head
with an affectionate murmur. They had been married for thirty-
some years.

Our meeting over tea soon led to an invitation back to dinner.
On that occasion, I was, in manner of speaking, initiated into the
family when his father played a prank on me. Without me looking,
Dudley had substituted two raw eggs for look-alike canned peach
halves coated in heavy syrup in my dessert bowl. When I stuck
my spoon into my first "peach," yellow swirls of yolk bled into the
"syrup." From the way everyone hooted at once, I knew that the
whole family must have been in on the joke. The implication that
they must have discussed it and decided I would be game gave me
so much joy that I laughed the loudest of all.

The happy togetherness Peter and his family bestowed on me
drew further into the spotlight the baffling question of why, then,
he never asked me on a proper date. Not for the first time, my roommate and I dissected this fraught situation. Did he have a secret

romance with a girl that his parents either did not know about or disapproved of? Had he been pledged at birth to the daughter of a war buddy who had saved his father's life? Was he gay?

Gradually, a potential explanation, if not an excuse, for Peter's tight-lipped avoidance of dating came to light, though it didn't come from him. Early on he had told me that he was passionate about ballroom dancing, that he participated in competitions, and that it took a lot of time. Now I got word from friends that he had been seen more than once at university dances with the same woman, who had long blonde hair and was an excellent dancer. But if I had spies out, so did he. He teasingly told me one Monday morning that one of his friends had seen me at a dance with another man the Friday before. I cringed. If I had been seen out with a tall, handsome partner who doted on me, I might not have minded. However, I was actually on an awful blind date with a guy who had worn yesterday's shirt and couldn't dance to save his pocket protector. While Peter's enquiry about my social life presented an opening for me to ask about his dance partner, I didn't take it. Neither did he volunteer any information. The next day, as usual, we took another long, delicious walk together after class.

Michael Gazzaniga points out that when we do not have enough cues to explain a situation, we very seldom say, "I don't know what is going on." Instead, "the human tendency to find order in chaos" causes our brains to fill in conspicuous gaps or loose ends so that "everything [fits] into a story and [is] put into a context." Gazzaniga calls the brain process that tends to confabulate rather than accept discrepancies *the interpreter*. It is located in the left hemisphere. The right hemisphere, in contrast, is utterly truthful. It "always choose[s] the option that has occurred the most frequently in the past." It insists on including information that doesn't make sense.

Gazzaniga has been studying the separate functions of the left and right brains for over half a century. His research subjects are people who had undergone surgery to sever the corpus callosum, "the superhighway of neurons connecting the halves of the brain," to obtain relief from epilepsy. After surgery, their left and right hemispheres are unable to communicate with each other. Accordingly, Gazzaniga designed tests to determine the function of each half in the composition of a narrative. In one test, he erected a barrier between the patient's eyes and placed separate objects or pictures in each visual field, thereby delivering simultaneous images to the left and right hemispheres. Gazzaniga explains that "[e]ach hemisphere was shown four small pictures, one of which related to a larger picture also presented to that hemisphere." The large picture shown to the left hemisphere portrayed a snowstorm, the right-hemisphere picture a bird claw.

> The patient had to choose the most appropriate small picture… [T]he right hemisphere—that is, the left hand—correctly picked the shovel for the snowstorm; the right hand, controlled by the left hemisphere, correctly picked the chicken to go with the bird's foot. Then we asked the patient why [his] left hand—or right hemisphere—was pointing to the shovel. [Since language production occurs in the left hemisphere, the answer originated on that side.] But because [the left hemisphere] could not know why the right hemisphere was doing what it was doing, it made up a story about what it could see—namely, the chicken. It said the right hemisphere chose the shovel to clean out a chicken shed.

In his book *Who's in Charge?*, Gazzaniga relates this research to the interpreter function: "the left hemisphere did not say 'I don't know,' which truly was the right answer...It confabulated, taking cues from what it knew and putting them together in an answer that makes sense."

Reflection on Dementia Notebook entry of 10-28-2011

You are downstairs getting dressed. On the bed you lay out a sartorial assemblage: turquoise-tinted black jeans, black shoes, your turquoise and black zebra-striped T-shirt, the turquoise earrings your neighbor Ann had given you when you lived on Supernal Way. But first, underwear. When you turn back from the closet, you wonder what earrings will work with the outfit. From your jewelry drawer you select the silver-and-black earrings. When you put them with the outfit, you notice that you had already selected another pair. Oh, well. But look how nicely your unwitting second choice evokes the zebra stripes of the T-shirt. There was a *reason* your brain did not stick with your first pick: your memory was triggered by the T-shirt's pattern because it had over the years stored such interesting stuff about zebras in its archives. *Equus quagga quagga.* A zebra species of which only the front half was camouflaged. In the albumen print of a lone mare that lived in Amsterdam's Artis Magistra zoo during the 1880s, the subject's posture of defeat resembles that of a specimen of *Equus asinus* that is known even to preschoolers, Eeyore, when he tries to think where he might have left his tail. The mare's stare is as spaced out as Sancho Panza's no-name donkey known only by an attribute, *rucio*, or dappled, a mental link whose farmyard connotations predisposes my mind's eye to envisage a silver-gray beast of burden patterned with golden circles of light, as if the clock struck once upon a midnight while she was dreaming under a moonlit tree. The hind part of the mare bears reddish brown and white bands like those that might be achieved by the geometric play of light and shadow through the bars of a prison.

Okay, another try, this time sans emotive constructions. Fact is that the coats of *Equus quagga quagga*; the modern zebra, *Equus quagga*; and the donkey, *Equus asinus*, all derive from the monkey business of that god who throws dice about whom Einstein wanted to know nothing, though Darwin secretly loved him: through a play of genetic replication over the millennia, the markings that used to camouflage the hind parts of the Urmother of all three species were retained by the zebra, half erased in the quagga, and completely erased in the donkey. In 1883, when it behooved the gambling god to recall the Amsterdam mare to Holy Headquarters, he performed an even more encompassing erasure: the mare had been the last of her breed, the only remaining representative of the subspecies on Earth. Since at the time the term *quagga* applied to any zebra found in southern Africa, however, no one noticed until the next century.

———————

Our second year of university threw Peter and me together for even more hours each day than the first. We had two required courses together, chemistry and maths, as well as *two* three-hour labs per week. Our test schedules, too, were almost exactly the same. We were together almost every daylight hour. Other than the fact that he had once invited me to a movie and I had invited him to a dance at my hostel, occasions on which we had held hands and snuck a quick kiss or two, our relationship remained essentially the same.

I tried to convince myself that all Peter and I might ever have would be a great friendship. How long, though, would such a friendship last once we graduated? Was it worth the daily torture of being around him while knowing he did not have the same long-term longing for me as I had for him? I decided not to mess with the part of our relationship that was working, but at the same time, to expend some of my emotional resources on the wider world. Not that my options were all that stellar. A rugby player I'll call Jaco, who had dated one of my classmates in high school, ran into me on campus. I had no idea that he even knew me, but somehow he did and he recognized me. Jaco asked me on a date, and we had a great time. More dates followed. Pretty soon we were kissing and cuddling. By the time the second semester of my second year was over, we were seeing quite a bit of each other. I would again spend the vacation in Pretoria, working for my scholarship and staying in a boarding house near the university. (Peter, again, would have a holiday with his extended family in Cape Town.) Being in Pretoria made it possible for Jaco and I to see each other more frequently, but more time with Jaco hastened my realization that he would never be a serious candidate for my heart.

I might very well have worked up the nerve to end things with Jaco were it not that I suddenly found myself homeless. For reasons I still don't understand, my landlady one day gave my room to a previous tenant who suddenly showed up demanding it back. When I came home after work, my belongings had been tossed on the bed and floor of a smaller and darker room at the back of the house. While I was still surveying my possessions in a stunned state, Jaco arrived for our date. He was much more loudly indignant than I had been, urging me to load my stuff in his car and walk away that very evening. That would have been very satisfying, except that I would not have a roof over my head. No problem, Jaco insisted, he would take me home to his parents' house, where he lived, and they would put me up for the night. Giving in to the short-term gratification of telling my landlady where she could stick her room, I agreed. At his house, his mother was unfazed at my unannounced arrival. She gave me the spare room and I settled in for the night, at least. His lovely and utterly gracious family insisted that I stay a while and not rush into a new place. I was to have dinner with them every night, which I did. With Jaco as my chauffeur and bodyguard, I found a new place to rent within a week.

Having seen a new side to my rugby player, I was having fun with him again. Besides, it would have been very bad manners to stop seeing such a kind boyfriend. I was shallow enough, though, to follow up on a more thrilling option that arose. One of the graduate assistants in my physics lab, whom I'll call John, was also working at the Atomic Energy Board, and we got to know each other on the long bus ride to and from work. John was interesting and attractive, and we had a certain chemistry. Even though he had told me early on that he had a fiancée, he invited me to coffee and I accepted. He was a great conversationalist who also played the violin and told me he sometimes seriously considered giving up his science career to become a professional musician. Despite the fact that his juxtaposition of talents twanged my heartstrings, I decided that being friends would be safe. We continued meeting and talking in public places.

My relationships with both Jaco and John continued when classes started and I was back at the hostel. Whether Peter had heard about my male companions, or maybe even spotted me with one of them, I did not know. On a very subtle level, though, he was paying me more attention. Our hands and arms brushed so much it couldn't be random—we had both, after all, studied basic statistics—and he did wacky things along the lines of his father's prank. One day in class, for example, he drew a cartoon on the back of my hand, which, of course, entailed holding my hand. I acted pretend angry, but underneath churned the real anger I already harbored toward him for playing loose and fast with my emotions. We still walked home as usual; I am not an ultimatum kind of person.

That evening after dinner at the hostel, the PA system echoed through my floor: "Gerda Steenekamp, front door." To my astonishment, there stood Peter. "I'm sorry I wrote on your hand," he said. "I've come to wash it off." Only then did I notice that he had a towel flung over his shoulder and carried a bar of soap. I couldn't help but laugh—and submit to yet another handholding in sheep's clothing.

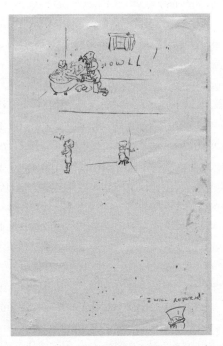

Peter's cartoon after the hand-washing episode, 1968

Over a number of coffees it proved that it was John, however, who had fallen in love with me. I had at least a crush on him, a mutual state of affairs of which we were both aware despite our ongoing impeccable behavior because of his fiancée. If it hadn't been for her, I might have given my emotions free rein. I was physically attracted to him and our minds strongly resonated. The labile center around which this maelstrom was spiraling, of course, could not hold. One day he invited me to tea at his house rather than to coffee in a restaurant. There he declared his attraction to me, told me that he and his fiancée were going through a difficult time. I did not need a second cup of tea to think anything through. Having any part in a potential breakup was not a burden with which I could live. I urged him in the strongest terms not to make any decisions that figured me in. We agreed not to see each other again.

(Reader, he married her. Fifteen years or so later, our children attended the same elementary school in Johannesburg.)

Having almost burnt my fingers in that conflagration, I stopped seeing Jaco as well, for good measure.

Maybe partly as a result of my conscience-clearing sweep, something seemed to be changing between Peter and me, and so it happened that somewhere between the agony of a three-hour Saturday morning chemistry exam one week (on Lewis's theory that the exchange of electron pairs between two solutions on opposite ends of the pH scale results in a *dative electron bond*) and a maths exam the next week (on L'Hopital's rule for detecting forbidden limits such as $0/0$ or ∞/∞), Peter and I started to study together—at his family's dining room table.

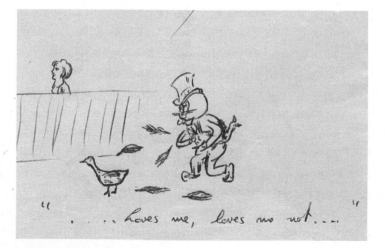

Peter's cartoon while we were studying together, 1969

What is there to report about two heads, often bent over the same book, trying to fathom strange new vocabularies deep into the night? What is there to explain about a kiss? Another kiss? An exploration of bodies? Maybe just one clarification is needed: Peter, too, had done important emotional housework before we started studying together. He had stopped competitive dancing and broken up with his blonde partner, who had, in fact, been his girlfriend. (Reader, she, too, loved well. The blonde girl had really never been my rival—rather, a kindred soul. When I met her forty years after she and Peter had broken up, she had spread goodness and healing in South Africa as a physician for many decades. Now, together with her beloved partner of twenty-some years, she is facing her own deteriorating health with honesty and fortitude. Together they agreed she will forgo further medical treatment for her breast cancer.)

I was almost eighteen, he nineteen, when we officially started going steady. For my first birthday that we celebrated together, he gave me a pair of white sandals, an item I had casually mentioned once. For no special occasion, he soon afterward gave me a ring: a sparkling, pea-sized oval of peridot, the soft green of spring grass, set in gold, with the bottom half of its egg delineated in tiny garnets. It was not an engagement ring, and I wore it on my right hand. When we mutually decided to become engaged on the day of our graduation ceremony—when my parents would be in town— that was the only ring I wanted. After a dinner at his parents' house that included my parents, he ceremonially removed the ring from my right hand and slipped it onto the customary finger on the left.

Over the years Peter's odd behavior at the start of our relationship made more sense. I came to realize that, for Saunders men, "going steady" is equivalent to mating for life. They had to be very, very sure before making what they saw as an unbreakable commitment. Examples abound. Peter's parents met when they were both only seventeen and never looked at another man or woman after that. Cliff and Ria met as neighbors when she was ten and he four-teen, and they started going steady in high school. Our son, New-ton, would continue the tradition. Like Peter and I, he and Cheryl started dating exclusively when he was nineteen and she eighteen.

Reflection on Dementia Field Notes 9-27-2013

In the lead-up to my sixty-fourth birthday, which was yesterday, I have been thinking a lot about *until death do us part*. If I have any fear of death, it is that it will not be timely enough to avoid the point when I will no longer recognize the people I love. As a friend of mine says when we speak about our mothers and grandmothers, "Old women never die." Men in my and Peter's families seem to die early. Both my and Peter's mothers had decades of widowhood. Since I experience their last years from a distance, with only short visits in person, I look elsewhere to learn about the dailiness of getting really old. Here in Roberta Street, we have two sets of neighbors who are living the ideal most of us have for our marriages or other long-term relationships: growing old together. The couple living diagonally across the road from us are both in their eighties, each coping with serious, physical, age-related illnesses, but are of sound mind. They regularly affirm to each other—sometimes while I'm visiting—their mutual love and gratitude. Our straight-across neighbors, Bob and Diane, are no pictures of physical health either, but for them, I believe, their biggest challenge is that Bob's mind and personality have been destroyed in a series of strokes. Diane is now in her late seventies, Bob a year or two younger.

Bob and Diane were married fifty years ago when Bob, just back from the Korean Mop Up, or clearing the country of remaining enemy troops, was touring the West with a soldier buddy and met Diane during a stop in Salt Lake City. This is a glimpse of what Diane has told me about their life together: Their marriage has been good, with a lot of jokes and laughter. They have two sons, both in Utah. Their younger, Randy—now in his fifties—suffered a brain aneurism in his thirties, functions at about the level of a four-year-old, and lives in a care center nearby. Bobbie, the older son, is their go-to family when it comes to health crises and house repairs. However, he lives some distance away and is employed in construction, where pay equals presence.

Since Bob's first massive stroke, Diane has spent at least twenty hours per day in the house with a husband who has no conversation and does not know the difference between day and night, making for an erratic sleep pattern. Bob constantly needs help with toileting, bathing, dressing, feeding, and staying safe. Diane stepped into this demanding caretaker role directly from her job of cleaning houses three days a week, an activity and income she had to give up three years ago when she became a full-time caregiver. Because of Bob's military service, his medical care is handled through the Veterans Health Administration (part of the VA). The VA provides an afternoon's respite care for Diane every second week. Other than the approximately eight hours per month that she has free to have her hair cut or go to her own doctor appointments, she is constantly in charge of Bob in a house with double-locked doors to prevent him from indulging his *wanderlust*.

Every second Sunday, Randy visits for the day. Diane keeps him and Bob busy by asking for their help in the garden. Randy is great at mowing the lawn. When it comes to other tasks, though, father and son need full-time guidance, which they don't necessarily follow. Once when I walked over while the family was out in their front yard, Diane watched in exasperation as they both attacked the rose bushes with pruning clippers. "With both of them at it," she said with a wry smile, "soon there will be only sticks left."

I love and admire Diane. There is no doubt in my mind that she is living out her marriage promises with love, devotion, and an intact sense of humor. And that there is great beauty and dignity in that.

While I have no doubt that Peter, too, will take ever-increasing care of me as my dementia worsens, is that what I want? Would he want me to do that for him in a reverse of our circumstances? Haven't we both always considered a death of the mind as a sufficient reason to hasten the moment when "death do us part"?

———————

Libido is likely one of Freud's most misunderstood terms—in everyday language it conjures up the sexual drive, particularly when it goes overboard. In psychoanalytical terms, though, libido is the energy we have for not only sexual love but all life-affirming psychic activity. To function as a human being, some part of the libido must be directed inward, that is, we must love ourselves before we can love anyone or anything else. Pouring all one's libido onto others can lead to not only psychic but also physical collapse. According to the Alzheimer's Association, "an older adult caring for another with dementia has a 60 percent chance of dying before the person they're taking care of because of the stress."

The Aquarian age that dawned with Peter's and my upside-down encounter under the desktop has resulted in a forty-eight-year relationship thus far, forty-five of them in the long haul of marriage. Our coming together engendered two wondrous material manifestations for whose coming-into-being we claim credit: our children. They, in turn, have expanded our being with grandchildren: Kanye, now almost eight years old, Aliya almost five, and Dante two. They are my *memento vivere*, or "remember to live."

When not going gaga over our children's remarkable parenting skills and our grandchildren's charm, Peter and I still pursue our own intellectual passions. He is the holder of eighty-seven US patents related to encryption and other identity-safeguarding technologies in the financial industry. Five times during the past six years, he has been honored as a Utah genius. Now that retirement has freed up his time, he is devoting himself to pursuits that extend the subject matter he knows into the personal realm—he is building a website centered on the under-the-hood mysteries of gathering enough money to retire, which includes philosophical reminiscences of how he and I have achieved that luxurious state (okay, to be real, let's say "frugally comfortable"), despite starting our lives over in our mid-thirties in a new country.

Over the years, our dancing has sadly been curtailed by the fact that ballroom dances of European origin have now become the quaint pastime of an earlier age. Even Latin dancing favors reggaeton, a blend of Latin and Caribbean music executed in the style of rap and hip-hop, and now almost totally excludes the Latin classics of our youth. Besides, dancing at these clubs rarely starts before eleven p.m.—and we are no longer eighteen and nineteen. That leaves private dance lessons to keep up our skills, which we take when we can afford them. Absolutely free, though, is our twirling about the kitchen while making lunch or doing the dinner dishes or wherever else a charmed strain of the right notes vibrates the air.

In public, Peter and I apparently sometimes appear to be newly in love, prompting smiles or even comments from strangers. The other day, when holding hands and joking as usual, we went into the city-county building near our house to talk to a Social Security counselor. A woman behind the enquiry desk greeted us with, "I suppose you two are here to get a marriage license?" It felt mar-velous to show her our wedding rings and tell her that, over four decades earlier,

We sailed away, for a year and a day,
to the land where the bong-tree grows...
and hand in hand, on the edge of the sand,
we danced by the light of the moon,
the moon,
the moon,
We danced by the light of the moon.

Chapter Six

Of Madness and Love II

At the start of 2015, seventy-eight-year-old Henry Rayhons, a nine-term Republican state legislator in Iowa, went on trial for third-degree felony sexual abuse for having sex with his wife of eight years. At the time of the alleged abuse, Donna Lue, whom Henry had met in a church choir and married in 2007, lived in a nursing home because of her advanced Alzheimer's. The *New York Times* reports a consensus among nursing home staff and the Rayhons's friends that they "had a loving, affectionate relationship." The charge against Mr. Rayhons does not allege that Mrs. Rayhons "resisted or showed signs of abuse." Care center staff report that "Mrs. Rayhons 'was always pleased to see Henry,'" who "visited his wife morning and evening, sometimes praying the rosary by her bed." The case, instead, hinges on the conviction of Mrs. Rayhons's daughter, Suzan Brunes, and the center's doctor, John Brady, that a person with advanced dementia is mentally unable "to give consent for any sexual activity."

Since Mrs. Rayhons's admission to the care center, Brunes had been concerned that Mr. Rayhons too often disturbed her mother's daily routine by taking her out to lunches with friends, church, or the funerals of friends and acquaintances. She requested that the nursing home assess Mrs. Rayhons's mental state. Upon being tested by her family doctor and a social worker at the center, Mrs. Rayhons scored zero on the test administered, because she was "unable to recall the words 'sock,' 'bed' and 'blue.'" Their conclusion was that Mrs. Rayhons could no longer consent to sex and, therefore, presumably no longer needed the privacy of her own room. She was moved to a double room. A few days later her roommate complained that she had heard "sexual noises" during one of Mr. Rayhons's visits. Suzan Brunes complained to the staff. According to the *New York Times,* "Mrs. Rayhons was taken to a hospital and examined for sexual assault. The so-called rape kit, which the state processed months later, did not identify any signs of injury or proof of intercourse." By then, Brunes had already obtained custody of her mother, moved her to a different nursing home with a special dementia unit, and restricted Mr. Rayhons's visits.

Mrs. Rayhons died in August 2014 at the age of seventy-eight. The *New York Times* reports that "her husband was arrested soon after her funeral."

Mr. Rayhons's lawyer, backed by medical and psychiatric professionals, questioned the validity of the assessment used to deprive the Rayhonses of their right to have sex, since "no widely used method exists for assessing the ability to consent to intimate relations. One obstacle: Dementia's symptoms fluctuate. Patients may be relatively lucid in the morning and significantly impaired in the afternoon." Mr. Rayhons's legal team also contended that "physical intimacy can benefit dementia patients…calming agitation, easing loneliness and possibly aiding physical health." Daniel Reingold, chief executive of the Hebrew Home at Riverdale, in the Bronx, which pioneered a "sexual rights policy" for residents in 1995, says that "touch is one of the last pleasures we lose." Given that aging and restriction to a long-term care facility cause "loss of independence, loss of friends, loss of ability to use your body, why would we want to diminish [physical intimacy]?"

These experts do not dispute the inability of a person in a vegetative state to consent to sex. However, dementia patients often retain considerable awareness even though they are unable to manage money, discern time, or recognize children. Gayle Doll, director of the Center on Aging at Kansas State University, believes that though "persons with dementia might not assent with words," they can still indicate a desire for touch and other sexual activity "with body language or facial expression." Mr. Rayhons's team therefore argued that people with dementia should not be deprived of "the capacity for self-determination and intimate relationships."

Dementia Field Notes

7-10-2012

When I went to a precheck for my colon surgery, I parked between an SUV and a shoulder-high wall. When I returned, someone was waiting for my parking spot, but I thought she was too close. I waved her back, and she retreated, but it wasn't enough. I motioned again, and she moved another inch. Still feeling cramped, I reversed, but when I turned I banged into the SUV. I got such a fright that I reversed and hit the concrete wall.

I wrote the SUV owner a note, called Peter. I told him our car was okay and I would drive back.

Bottomless dread.

Back home, I told Peter I was no longer going to drive. Since it was the day I usually took our elderly neighbors shopping, I went over to tell them I would not be taking them that day or again in the future. I could not bring myself to tell anyone else. It wasn't so much the driving, but rather the change in what I think of as a core of my self: helping other people.

7-16-2012

On Saturday morning I made a statement about not driving: I went shopping. By bus. At Fashion Place Mall. An hour there and an hour back. Nothing like being one of the elite on the bus who are not toothless, homeless, in a wheelchair, or on oxygen to take my mind off myself. Nothing to make my troubles seem trivial like the disproportionately large number of African Americans, Native Americans, and Hispanics awakening my racial privilege.

12-31-2012

Returning by bus from Fashion Place in the late afternoon, I inadvertently got off twelve blocks too soon, a mistake I realized only after I had crossed the street. Since the temperature was nineteen degrees and the next bus due in half an hour and there was no shelter, I swallowed my pride and called Peter to come get me.

After Peter and I were married, we each added a year or so of post-bachelor study. Then followed six years of acquiring professional jobs, a house, furniture, a sound system, and a six-week trip to Asia. Our first child, Marissa, was born during the seventh year of our marriage. After a day of hard labor, she slid into the world, and I impatiently strained to get a glimpse of her while she was still tied to me. Peter described her as "a beautiful little girl with red lips." Since she was distressed and cold after the umbilical cord wrapped around her neck toward the end of a long labor, I only got to hold her for a few moments before she was taken away to be warmed in a covered, heated crib. I had planned to put her to my breast within the first minutes after her birth—as the books said—and had a sense of something far worse than disappointment when I was denied the chance. Giving her back to the nurse was like giving up an arm.

Fortunately our daughter soon rallied, and I was able to hold and nurse her. When I wasn't holding her, Peter was. In between, she slept in a crib beside my bed. Although I was exhausted, I fought sleep because closing my eyes would mean I could not see her. I was in love. All I wanted to do was hold her against my naked body, stroke her face and tummy, kiss the top of her head and her little pink hands, lick her toes.

I was headlong, hoplessly, ecstatically in love.

Two and a half years after Marissa's birth, Newton burst into our lives, his scrunched-up face yelling annoyance that it took us so long to get him out. I was able to put him to my breast and hold him and love him, as besotted as I was with my firstborn, with his warmth against my skin, his greedy rooting for my nipple, and his feisty, "masculine" way of thrusting his little arms and legs into my torso and lap when I held him. He, too, stayed in a crib by my bed. Since my labor with him was even longer and harder than with Marissa, I drifted off into sleep soon after Peter had gone home to tell Marissa and Ouma Raaitjie about our little boy. Before I had fallen into a deep sleep, I was awakened by a choking sound. When I pulled Newton from his crib, he was blue, not breathing.

What friends would later call my "hyena mommy mode" kicked in. I shouted for help, all the while wobbling to the nurse's station as fast as someone with episiotomy stitches could hope to do. The nurse on duty rushed toward me, reaching me not a second too soon. I put my baby in her outstretched hands, fainted, and crumpled to the floor. The next time I knew what was going on, Peter was telling me that Newton was okay. He had aspirated some fluids during the labor, the nurses had cleaned out his airways, and they would be observing him in the baby room for the night, though they would still bring him to me to nurse. My doctor took my fainting spell as an indication that the transfusion he had been considering in light of my blood loss was now inevitable. I would be transfused the next day.

As it sadly sometimes goes in medical situations, the intended cure proved worse than what led to it. I turned out to be one of the approximately 0.003 percent of people who suffer anaphylactic shock from a plasma protein in the blood component. About ten minutes into the transfusion, I told the nurse by my side that my feet felt funny. I had never in my life been the object of a flurry of activity of the magnitude that followed. The last thing I remember was a circle of faces around my bed. After the loss of consciousness, after the antihistamines, the oxygen, the adrenaline, and the steroids, I needed additional blood even more than at the outset. The next day, I was again transfused, this time starting with an antihistamine. Despite my restored blood volume, I was really sick. It took an additional three days before I could take my baby home. The worst effect of the dramatic episode, though, is that I did not feel any love for my son. I might as well have been holding the baby of a neighbor's niece from Windhoek.

Whatever happened to my brain after the anaphylactic shock must have affected my facial recognition pathway—fortunately only temporarily. When I discovered the Capgras phenomenon, the descriptions of patient responses sounded eerily like my own when I felt a big blank about Newton. He sure looked like the baby I loved right after he was born, but why, then, did I feel nothing?

In what I think of as an example of one of the central claims of existentialism, "existence precedes essence"—the idea that a human life does not have meaning in itself but that we create our own significance through our conscious acts—I went through the motions of caring for my son once we were home. In the same way that faking a smile can improve one's mood—as shown by psychologist Paul Ekman—my faking of loving maternal behavior started upping my oxytocin levels and within a few weeks I was romancing my son in the same way I had his sister before him.

To this day, my son has never stopped lighting my life. Whenever I see him or talk to him, I still feel the awe-filled openness of the love that slowly blossomed for him in my soul, a love that, to my feminist chagrin, warrants Freud's statement that a mother's relation to her son "is altogether the most free from ambivalence of all human relationships." My redemption as a feminist lies in the fact that Freud's words also perfectly match my feelings for my daughter.

In a letter he wrote for my sixty-fourth birthday Peter says,

> I want you to be there when anything important happens to me to say some of those beautiful words of yours. Although I really hope we die together at the same moment and in the same place, if I am the one to die first I want you to speak some of your words to our family and friends. My nitrogen, carbon, oxygen, and hydrogen molecules will vibrate just a little faster when the energy of your words reach them while they burn furiously in the furnace.

Although Peter and I are not queasy about talking, joking, and sometimes being sad about a time when one or both of us will no longer be, it is not death we have on our minds most of the time. We are really into living. And *living* for older people, much more so than younger people might imagine or even want to know, includes sex. For you voyeurs out there—and I count myself in your company—I refer you to articles such as "Sex and the Seniors: Survey Shows Many Elderly People Remain Frisky" or "Sex and the Senior Citizen: How the Elderly Get It On" for summaries of "the most comprehensive sex survey ever done among 57- to 85-year-olds in the United States." The results show that Peter and I are by no means the only sexagenerians who follow the prescription "use it or lose it."

As far as telling tales out of the bedroom goes, I will reveal only two things: (1) as in the days when we were trying to make babies, we have to have sex by the calendar—one of us has to be off certain medications and the other on additional ones to jump-start those hoary neurons into squirting their dopamine; and (2) to achieve the *jouissance* that was there for the taking half a century ago whenever one of us was hot to trot, now, like many of our peers, we "have to work harder at it." But we're retired; we have time.

There really isn't an age limit to having sex. As long as people have access to sex partners (or whatever else turns them on), they will keep on having sex. In the absence of partners, they will pleasure themselves—a practice cheered on health websites for seniors. In keeping sexually active until a great age, people in long-term relationships have an edge—they are most likely to have someone around to have sex with when the hormones start to "vibrate just a little faster." Interestingly, "people who stay in their first marriages instead of getting divorced and remarried, often have more sex," says an article titled "Married Couples' Sex Lives Rebound—After 50 Years, Study Finds."

In a Daily Beast section titled "In the Sheets," Barbie Nadeau writes that "if the thought of two nude octogenarians tangled up in the sheets doesn't make you cringe, chances are you have reached a level of maturity when sex after a certain age seems like a pretty good idea." I, now, am "mature" enough to hope that my Ouma Truia and Oupa Carel had sex throughout their sixty-three years of marriage.

Dementia Field Notes

04-24-2014

Last week Diane took her annual break to visit her sisters in Mesquite, Nevada—a five-hour drive. Ahead of time, she had booked Bob into a care center—the VA pays for it. Their son Bobbie would take him there as soon as Diane had left. The previous year Bob got very anxious when she left, so this time Bobbie lured him for a ride in his truck so she could sneak away. Their destination: the care center.

The next evening, Bob walked away from the center—his wristband failed to set off the door alarm. The night staff discovered his absence at midnight, called 911. Peter and I heard about it through a missing person's call in the morning. By then there were cops at their house, about to do a door-to-door search. They organized the neighbors who had shown up to search in different directions. Peter and I drove and walked our assigned area, but no luck. Bob was found seventeen hours after he escaped, six miles from the center. The person who spotted him thought he was dead: He was completely still, leaning semi-upright on an electrical box. The paramedics established that he had merely fallen into an exhausted sleep.

In the afternoon, Bob arrived home in an ambulance, followed by Bobbie in his truck. Bob was too weak to walk, so two paramedics walked him up the porch stairs. He immediately started calling for Diane. However, she was still on the road—her sister could only start driving home in daylight, because she had lost her night vision. When Diane arrived an hour or two after Bobbie had tucked Bob into bed, she vowed never to leave him again.

On March 26, 1971, Peter's and my wedding day, I rose at first light. I had slept at my parents' house. So had my friend Bettie, who was famous in our hostel for her flair with hair. When the alarm went off at five a.m., we both awakened tired and bedraggled after a night on the living room carpet with only a pillow and a blanket as bedding. My parents' house was bursting with relatives who had not come for the wedding, but came to assist my ninety-something Kalahari oupa, who was staying with my parents while Ouma Truia was in a hospital in Pretoria after a serious car accident. Bettie and I, being the halest and heartiest of the guests, were the best candidates for the living room floor. To make matters worse, I had gone to sleep with rollers in my hair.

I had arrived at my parents' house later than planned the night before, and I still had to finish sewing my wedding veil. The Henning family had come over from Iowa and were staying in our apartment. While stitching a lace edging onto the gossamer white fabric of my headpiece—the same material out of which I had made my wedding dress—I chatted with Al, Dorothy, and my American sisters. Distracted and in a hurry to get to my parents' place, I accidentally cut a slit near the edge of the veil. Dorothy immediately became my mom again, as she had been during the year in Iowa. She talked me out of the panic that made me wring my hands, took the sewing from my lap, and completed not only the edging, but also darned the slash. The next morning, before I had even washed my bleary eyes, I quickly reassured myself that the veil and the rest of my wedding regalia were in good order and that what we would today call a "wardrobe malfunction" had only been the stuff of my floor-sleeping nightmares. Everything was in order. I was ready for my makeover.

During the hour or so it took Bettie to pile my shoulder-length hair on top of my head, she remained as unperturbed as if she were merely calculating the Fourier coefficients of a non-harmonic equation. When she was done, she coaxed a few tendrils from the massed curls to frame my face. Then it was time to step into my dress: a high-waisted style with a softly gathered skirt falling to the floor, its bottom eighteen inches adorned with lace insets. Its unlined sleeves were full on the upper arm and, from the elbow to the wrist, as skin-hugging as long evening gloves. Once I had twirled around in front of the mirror to Bettie's approving oohs and ahs, all that remained was for Bettie to fix my veil, somewhere at the back among the poufy curls, with a spray of frangipani. Since I had decided to be a "modern" bride, the veil was merely decorative and would not cover my face. Today there was to be no screen, no matter how fine, between me and the wondrous world.

After a seven a.m. solo photo shoot at a park where Peter and I had made many memories since we had met, I headed for the church. My father was waiting at the main door. When the wedding march started, we followed the flowergirls (eight-year-old Tertia and a cousin) and maids of honor (Lana and my American sister Joyce) down the aisle. My father kissed me, shook Peter's hand, and held on to my shoulder until Peter pulled me toward him. My almost-husband's look of awe and tenderness when I was close enough for our eyes to meet was poetry made flesh: "i carry your heart with me (i carry it in / my heart)."

The Afrikaans Dutch Reformed ceremony that followed was canonical, the words so familiar that they took on the calming tone of a benificent incantation. The only nontraditional aspect of our church union would be Peter's ringing "Ja" to the requisite questions, a response that would draw suppressed laughter from the participants, breaking the tight-lipped silence that usually reigned in Afrikaans churches.

After a family and couples photo session, Peter and I finally arrived at our reception. The already assembled guests waved and smiled as we strolled hand-in-hand across the Mulders' green lake of lawn, interspersed with islands of native trees. On a jungle gym along our path, the young guests were doing gravity-defying, legs-in-the-air topsy-turvies so that my flowergirls' lilac dresses folded like jacaranda bells over their heads. On the patio, where the guests were already at their tables, the trellised bougainvillea radiated purple-red joy onto everyting. Nodding and waving like royalty, Peter and I walked among family and friends to our seats, admiring our host Tant Lettie's—a longtime friend of Peter's family—golden touch.

Each table flaunted a bowl of freshly squeezed orange juice at the center, a yellow sun surrounded by an asteroid belt of pineapples, grapes, bananas, and apples. Behind the main table, where Peter and I would sit with our parents, a buffet table was stacked with egg dishes, bacon platters, loaves of bread, bowls of fruit salad, and a tureen of coffee. Towering over the food was one of my mother's trademark giant flower arrangements, a cascade of rusty chrysanthemums, dark yellow Afrikaners, and light yellow carnations, all embedded in greenery Susanna had harvested from her own and her neighbors' gardens.

When the festivities ended around noon, Peter and I left for our honeymoon, the destination of which he had kept a secret until just a few days before I had to start my packing: a beach hotel in Durban. I changed from my wedding dress into a going-away outfit before we said our goodbyes. Lana had sewn the tight-fitting, calf-length cranberry-red suit as a wedding gift. Flitting among the guests so that the flared bottom of my skirt revealed about as much leg as a minidress, I felt fashionably louche and ready to be ensconced like a Proustian mistress in our hotel, the Oyster Box, an establishment whose name I would only properly appreciate once I left behind the world of science for the unblushing frontiers of feminist literary criticism and historicize the double entendres of our honeymoon lodgings. At that moment, though, my libido was not intent upon deciphering any intellectual tidbits whatsoever. Feeling as decidedly unfeminist as the never-married biblical observer of two millennia earlier, Mrs. Saunders, six hours married, fit the 1 Corinthians 7:34 bill: "she that is married careth for the things of the world, how she may please her husband."

Dementia Field Notes

2-16-2013

My second neuropsychological test results came in the mail while we were in Chicago, gone to help Marissa and Adam stock the freezer and wash the baby clothes in time for their first baby's birth—my third grandchild! Back home, I found the neuropsychological report in the huge box of mail our neighbor Diane had collected for us. I read it, but could not bring myself to write anything about it until now—over two weeks later.

Right after the test, while debriefing with my neuropsychologist—I'll call her DeeDee—I had great confidence in the outcome of the working memory test, the one where I had to remember the four sets of words. During my test two years ago, I had demonstrated only "average learning ability." Since I had learned during that test cycle that the sixteen words came in semantic clusters—giraffe zebra squirrel cow, cabbage celery onion spinach—it felt as if I were doing better the second time round. To my disappointment, though, the results show that my overall score this time was worse than at age sixty-one.

The report's fine print explains my lower overall score. Even though I knew the words came in four categories, after most repeats I could remember only three categories. I remember saying, "I know there is one I haven't said yet," but could not come up with what it was. Together with the missing category all four of its words were lost. And this had been the section for which I'd had the highest hopes.

In the other sections my score had not gone downhill as much as I had expected based on how challenging they felt during the test. In the connect-the-numbers and build-the-diagram sections I had not made many mistakes, but my slowness lowered the scores. After I struggled through those sections, DeeDee must have seen how demoralized I was because she hinted that I might not want to do the math test this time. I was happy to leave it out. The report of two years ago already attested to the sorry state of my math skills.

What unnerves me most in both sets of test results, though, is the drop in my IQ since my last high school test. In my day, South African schools used the Wechsler scale, which is the same as the one DeeDee used. The results are therefore comparable, and the drop in my number precipitous.

Even though I know that IQ is nowadays regarded as too simplistic a measure of anyone's achievement potential and only tangentially related to life success, mine had always mattered to me. It stood for the academic prowess for which I was recognized as long as I can remember. When I was first tested in elementary school, it seemed that my score contributed to my parents' headtrip in regarding me as *ouderwets*, or fetchingly precocious. When I was older, it was something I knew was good about myself like my height and good skin and ability to stay calm. Now my IQ has become one of those things that I don't like: my sagging jowls, my slight limp from an old foot surgery, my wandering attention.

Until I have made peace with myself about this, I cannot talk about it with anyone. Not even Peter.

―――――――

Settling into the daily rhythms of life in a new city is challenging itself, but when the new city is also in a new country, finding those rhythms can take a while longer. Should our move have entailed a job or university course or some other anchoring environment for me as it did for Peter and our children, I might have found my niche with the same comparative ease that they did. However, without the appropriate visa I lacked the legal identity to participate in the kind of intellectual environments I had found exciting and challenging during my pre-parental years. For a while, I continued to embrace my identity as a "full-time mother," volunteering at my children's school, staging art and science events at our house, and facilitating my children's and our family's building of a social network. However, one can push one facet of her identity only so far and for so long: a year or two into our new life, I felt frustrated, unchallenged, and depressed. I did not love the self to which I had dwindled.

The first solution I attempted was to write. First, I wrote essay-style letters about our new life to update our family and friends in South Africa, then stories and a novel for children under the auspices of a mentor I found through a correspondence course in writing for children. After a year or two of this—and still no work visa in sight—I petitioned Utah senator Orrin Hatch for support in enabling me to enroll at the University of Utah as an in-state rather than a foreign student, thereby enabling me to afford the fees. I am unaware of the mechanism of my eventual acceptance at the U of U, but accepted I was. My initial goal of obtaining a Utah teacher certificate was soon eclipsed by the serendipitous publication of a story I had written in one of my classes, "Intro to Creative Writing," in a local magazine, *Utah Holiday*. I never did obtain that teaching certificate. Instead, particularly with the encouragement of one of my professors, I applied for a teaching fellowship in the master's program in creative writing and was accepted. After a year in the program, it seemed evident to me (and fortunately also to my

professors) that I should have applied for the direct track PhD program in creative writing. I obtained a transfer to that program, a
move that represents the major identity-forging experience of my
adult life. In addition to being an apartheid-shaped Afrikaner, sci-
entifically minded scholar and teacher, wife, mother, feminist, and
atheist immigrant, I now cloaked that self in a Gogolian overcoat
of philosopher/intellectual, an identity overlay that swelled my
being—like Akaky Akakievich Bashmachkin in his new coat—into
something "fuller, as if [I] were married."

In another vocabulary, I was again finding my voice.

On other ego fronts—in Freudian parlance—I was diversify-
ing my libidinal portfolio: In 1992, our whole family finally became
American citizens. With my PhD and citizenship in hand, I was eli-
gible to get a "real" job. Nevertheless, I stayed on for a year or two
at the U's English Department as an adjunct instructor. Eventually
I felt the pull of my duty to contribute a more equitable share to our
family's income. While still teaching part time, I tried a stint as a
technical writer at the U's Computer Science Department. Needing
a bigger challenge, I ventured into the business world, where, in
my seven-year career at three different companies, I was fortunate
enough to end up as one of two managers of a team of about forty
writers, programmers, and graphic artists that created training
materials for clients ranging from Rockwell Collins to Miller Beer
to Duke University's law school. The commercial world of business, however, was not for me. There, in the words of Luce Irigaray,
"the soul spends and is spent in the margins of capital."

In an odd throw of God's dice, an opportunity for me to return
to academics came during the screening of the 2002 film *Derrida*,
a biographical documentary of the eponymous French philosopher
who developed a mode of literary analysis known as deconstruc-
tion, which demonstrates the contradictions hidden in the founding
texts of Western philosophy. Also in the documentary's audience of

the who's who of literary critical aficionados in Salt Lake City was Kathryn Stockton, now a distinguished professor in the English Department of the U of U, who at the time served as the director of the Gender Studies Program. She invited me to apply for the about-to-be-vacant position of the program's associate director.

Doña Quixote: The rest, as we threadbare feminist literary connoisseurs like to say, is "herstory."

In April 2015, newspapers reported that former Iowa legislator Henry Rayhons was found not guilty of sexually abusing his wife. He had testified that "Donna and I would 'play.' She would reach in my pants and fondle me sometimes." He told the prosecutor, "I always assumed that if somebody asks for something, they have the capacity' to consent."

During his three and a half hours of testimony, Mr. Rayhons broke into tears ten times. "We just loved to be together," he said. "I treated her like a queen. She treated me like a king. I loved her very much. I miss her every day."

Reflection on Dementia Field Notes of 11-7-2011

Retired University of Utah faculty still have library privileges. Tracking down your wish list along the library's boustrophedon of call numbers, you also cherry-pick their next-door, upstairs, and downstairs neighbors: Michael Paterniti's *Driving Mr. Albert: A Trip across America with Einstein's Brain*; Jonah Lehrer's *Proust Was a Neuroscientist*; Barbara G. Walker's *Feminist Fairy Tales*; Edith Grossman's new translation of *Don Quixote*, with an introduction by Harold Bloom; René Daumal's *A Night of Serious Drinking*.

Setting out for home along the route you drove to school and work for twenty-some years, you float across the familiar suburb-scape, bobbing as leisurely as Einstein's brain in a Tupperware bowl in the trunk of a Buick Skylark. As you stop for a pedestrian crossing, your mother tongue asserts itself: *zebra oorgang*. Why did the zebra cross the solar system? Because it was immortalized as an image on the gold-plated disc affixed to the 1970s *Voyager* spacecraft, launched along with greetings in sixty human languages and the calls of the humpback whales.

Observing an orange-flag-wielding pedestrian, you think, "Whether the zebra crosses the road or the road crosses the zebra depends upon your frame of reference." For didn't South African scientists clone quaggas from tissue preserved from that Amsterdam mare—the first DNA of an extinct organism to be cloned and sequenced—and then selectively breed the plains zebra to produce a foal, Khumba,* whose coat coloration resembles that of quaggas? Einstein's topsy-turvy universe, like the one in which you suddenly find yourself. But yours is not comfortingly galactic. Uncanny, rather. You have stepped into a View-Master reel—"Hansel and Gretel"? Your cousin's *Don Quijote de la Mancha* with its tauntingly inexplicable foreign subtitles? Trees arch overhead. Stage left, a cottage slouches behind the trunks. Are you going east-west or north-south? Are these the trees near the gas station where you turn west, or the foresty tunnel you enter after already having turned? There are no street signs. The birds have eaten your breadcrumbs.

---

* Additional topsy-turviness: The foal was retroactively named Khumba, after the title character in a South African animated film by Triggerfish Animation Studios, after the scientific Quagga Project that created the real-life foal had died due to a lack of funding. "The Quagga Revival," as previously cited.

In the rearview mirror you note cars backed up behind you. *Dear Professor Einstein: I understand the world moves so fast, it in effect stands still.* A honk from the vehicle on your heels sets the others off. You cede the road, sidle almost onto the sidewalk. *Part of the time it seems a person is standing right side up; part of the time, on the lower side of the world, he stands on his head. And part of the time he sticks out at right angles and part of the time at left angles.* The aggrieved drivers pass, bestowing dirty looks. You sit with the engine running, waiting for—what? Baba Yaga in her speeding mortar fixing to scoot you along with her pestle? The *Moskva?*

Something from a witch's cauldron rises up your gullet. From your face, emotions sprout in warty patches. *I'm going to devour you alive. Your brain has dried up. You're a space cadet.* The European Space Agency will soon launch two spacecraft, the *Hidalgo* and the *Sancho*, to divert asteroids hurtling toward Earth.

An approaching semitruck blasts its troll breath from its overhead exhaust pipes, reminding you that the windmill you face is neither the size of Manhattan nor celestial. You have a scientific bent. Continue along this street and you will recognize something sooner or later. You are Doña Quixote crossing the equator in the Enchanted Boat. You are big nanny goat Gruff confronting your inner troll. *Up you jump.* You take a gap in the traffic, speed up like someone who knows where she's going. Soon the landscape will shift and you'll say, "Ah, there are those two houses with xeriscaped gardens right next to each other."

For a while Anytown, USA, keeps rolling by. But finally—a boxy two-story building differentiates itself from its look-alike neighbors: the dentist where Newton had his wisdom teeth out. *Trip-trap, trip-trap.* Just half a block to the Sizzler. *Up goes the troll. He goes SPLASH in the water.* Right angle, ten blocks to the light on 300 East. *Big nanny goat Gruff is over the bridge.* Left angle at the light, right angle at the blue house, right angle at Amit and Ruchika's. *The nanny goats Gruff have fun in the grass. They eat and eat. We like it here, they say.*

You stack the library books next to your two-seater couch. You sink into your side, lever up the footrest, cover your knees with the blanket Peter's mother had crocheted. Like Proust's madeleine, *this memory is but regret for a particular moment; your mom-in-law's treasured handcrafts are as fugitive as, alas, the years.* Your hand greedily clamps the top two books from your hard-won stash. You think of Albert Einstein's mother when his teachers announced the boy was *too stupid to learn.* She had him begin violin lessons. Remembering her later in life, Einstein would say, *A table, a chair, a bowl of fruit, and a violin; what else does a man need to be happy?* Before you settle on which book to open, your eyes fall on Peter, who is working on his laptop at the table.

> *Would it be reasonable to assume that falling in love is one of the stupid things one does while sticking out upside down on the bottom of the earth?*
> > *Sincerely,*
> > *Frank Wall*
>
> Dear Mr. Wall,
> *Falling in love is not at all the most stupid thing people do, but gravitation cannot be held responsible.*
> > *Sincerely,*
> > *Albert Einstein*

Glimmerings of the notion that mind and matter were very much connected had been flickering toward medical consciousness for centuries. Michael Gazzaniga regards eighteenth-century Austrian physician Franz Joseph Gall as the immediate forerunner of the modern "idea that different parts of the brain produce different mental functions" and its corollary that "injury to a specific part of the brain produce[d] deficits in a specific mental function." Unfortunately, Gall was also the father of phrenology, or the theory that the surface and shape of the skull revealed a person's abilities and character, resulting in the eventual tossing out of this crucial insight together with the pseudoscience he invented.

During the 1830s, French neurologist Marc Dax reported to the Academy of Sciences that three of his patients who had similar speech disturbances were found at autopsy to have similar left-hemisphere lesions. Since Dax was a provincial doctor, his findings did not impress the Parisian bigwigs. Thirty years later one of those bigwigs, Paul Broca, published an autopsy on a patient identified as Tan, since *tan* was the only word he was able to say. Having studied Tan's aphasia while he was alive, Broca traced his patient's communication deficits to a left-hemisphere lesion he found in his frontal lobe at autopsy. This brain region, named Broca's area, stands as the first surviving marker of the concept of mind/brain correlatives, without which contemporary neuroscience cannot exist.

A decade later, German surgeon Carl Wernicke discovered a correspondence between a lesion in the left temporal lobe and a second kind of aphasia, one that robs patients of their understanding of language while leaving them with the ability to utter nonsensical strings of words that retain some aspects of grammar. Wernicke's language area together with Broca's continue to serve as a key explanatory model for the variety and oddity of language losses incurred by stroke or other brain injuries.

Knowledge about the exact relationship between lesions and functional losses points to rehabilitation approaches most likely to succeed, foremost of which is "hit[ting] the injured brain hard with what it has lost, [namely] contact with its familiar, social environment." A 2005 brain imaging study proves what relatives and caretakers of people with dementia have long known: "the sound of a loved one's voice activated widely distributed circuits" in the brains of seriously brain-injured patients, and the most stimulating social environment possible leads to the highest possible levels of lucidity in old age, even in people who "have brains that appear riddled with Alzheimer's disease" or other dementia-type lesions. "Many of them remain social to the end, engaged in regular card games or debates with friends who make mental demands of them."

The same connection to a social environment is, of course, also crucial for those among the brain-damaged still lucky enough to be making mental demands on ourselves.

Dementia Field Notes

10-11-2015

Ever since Bob had gone to the VA hospice, Diane was too sick to visit him. Because of having the flu on top of emphysema, she could barely breathe and had to use oxygen all the time. There was no question of Bobbie taking Diane to see Bob, since she did not have a portable oxygen tank, only the stationary one with a long pipe for use at home. One day she told me she was better and off oxygen for a few hours during the day, and ready for me to take her on the bus to see Bob. We weren't even at the bus stop before she got heavier and heavier on my arm, and sank to the ground. I took her head on my lap and called her name while stroking her hair. She opened her eyes, but had no breath to speak. I called Peter; we took her to the emergency room. We stayed until Bobbie's wife could pick her up about two hours later.

To my astonishment, she was back home that afternoon. Bobbie was going to bring food and groceries and stay the night. When I popped in the next morning, he had left for work, but she had soup she could warm and said she was fine. When I checked on her after we had dinner, she was eating an orange cupcake. "Ah, dessert," I said.

"Oh, this is my dinner," Diane said. "I am too dizzy to fix myself something." I had some meat pie left from our dinner, so I took it over. From then onward, we have taken over dinner every day— she says it's enough for her for breakfast and lunch, too. Because of my upcoming trip to South Africa for my fiftieth Matric reunion, though, I worried that she would not manage when I was gone. With Diane's permission, I called Meals on Wheels and she was signed up. It starts only three days after I have left, however, but David and Lynda, who live next door to her, are going to take food over until Meals on Wheels kicks in. Peter, too, will check in every day.

The VA hospice reports that Bob's main daily activity is walking from window to window and door to door, looking to escape. When he gets tired, he gets into the nearest bed and pets the person already in it.

It is going on two weeks now since Bob and Diane have last seen each other. She asked me to help her call her doctor to prescribe a portable oxygen tank. She wants to be ready when Bobbie has time to take her to see Bob.

Doña Quixote: *Where are you going, Gertjie?*

Willeman: *There are no street signs. The birds have eaten your bread crumbs.*

Doña Quixote: *Willeman had his dogs.*

Gerda: *I have Peter.*

At our red front door, Doña Quixote stops. She is not yet allowed to enter. I alone cross the threshold, look for my dear, naughty little sweetheart. I find him in his half of our his-and-her chair. His computer lies closed on the coffee table. He has turned on his side, his head drooping toward the arm rest. His snore is rhythmic and loud. I have known him since I was seventeen and he nineteen; we met in physics class. I know what he will say, voice blurry with tenderness, when I tell him about the statistically meaningful downward migration of my IQ on the bell curve: "A table, a meat pie, a glass of wine, a hand to hold: what else does a man need to be happy?"

I let myself down gently, lever up the footrest, spoon up beside him. His shoulder pushes up a wave of his mother's crotchet blanket, and that is where I rest my head. He grunts, pets my leg. I think of the belugas' dissonant chatter as they follow the *Moskva* home, clots of sound overscored by the strings and winds of the orchestra. I think of the trills of their kin on the *Voyager* traversing the profound silence beyond the star that gave them life. How strange to the beings of those globular worlds the glissandos of the humpback whales.

Chapter Seven

Makeovers in Extremis

ON AUGUST 16, 2012, Marikana, the village near the farm where I grew up, garnered international infamy when the South African Police fired live ammunition on mineworkers striking for better pay. The action was carried out under the direction of the ruling ANC political party, the entity that had overthrown apartheid and now governs the country. The confrontation would be identified as "the deadliest security operation since apartheid was abolished." It would become known as the Marikana massacre.

The playing field on that spring day was far from level. As the miners congregated on the side of a hill amid the greening tufts of sweetgrass studded with pink patches of cosmos, a *sangoma*, or witchdoctor, anointed some of them with *muti*, or magical potions, "to protect them from police and make them immune to bullets." Other demonstrators carried *knobkerries* (clubs), *pangas* (machete-like knives), spears, and sticks. As the crowd of protesters grew, "hundreds of police backed by helicopters, armored vehicles and mounted units" started surrounding the assembled strikers with coils of barbed wire "with the aim of containing them to...disarm them more easily." Fearing that all escape routes would soon be cut off, a group of protesters broke away and rushed a police line. The police opened fire with automatic weapons. When the shooting stopped, thirty-four protesters lay dead and seventy-eight wounded. The police would later claim that they had been attacked with firearms. When all was over, police gathered five pistols and a truckload of "traditional weapons" from among the dead and immobilized.

When talking with American friends about the massacre, I found myself vacillating between two interlocking narratives, one depicting the idyllic time before the intrusion of unsettling politico-socioeconomic forces and the other directed to the recent eruption of violence. The longer I spoke, the more it became apparent to me that the seeds of today's violence were already, during my childhood, sprouting beneath the façade of apartheid-enforced peace.

Marikana, situated about seven miles from our farm, is where we obtained our library books; bought our groceries, vegetables, and newspapers; and, on certain Fridays when the delicacy was trucked in on smoking dry ice, ice cream. Marikana's main source of groceries and clothing was Katzenellenbogen Algemene Handelaars, the general store. Its owners were a Jewish family who did not live in the *platteland*, or country, but drove in every day from the larger town of Rustenburg. The store was known by all as *die Jood*, or the Jew. By the same logic, the Indian trader around the corner whose fabric store almost exclusively catered to black people, was known as *die Koelie*, or the Coolie. My cousin told me that when you walked by a Coolie, you should say, "Mohammed ate a pig." When I repeated this wisdom in front of my parents, they explained why the remark was an insult and forbade me to repeat it. When we did once go to *die Koelie* to buy fabric for saris to wear to our church women's international dinner, my mother greeted the owner with a handshake. It was the first time I had seen a handshake between a white and a dark-skinned person.

While *die Koelie* and the café had only one entrance for all races, *die Jood* had a separate entrance for blacks. The village library was for whites only. These details occurred to me only later in life. For a five-year-old white child, as for most white people in the farming district, apartheid was a presence so naturalized that one would be as likely to think about it as one's own breathing. Only through the lens of subsequent history did I come to understand that the village of my childhood must have been seething with black—not to mention Indian—anger. As a child, though, I accepted the blacks' obsequious lifting of hats and averted-eye greetings of "Môre, nonnie," or "Good morning, little Miss," as an ordinary part of life. The Setswana greeting that our house maid taught me often garnered me a broad smile and an enthusiastic response from people who suddenly looked like individuals rather than the interchangeable actors of my childhood.

"Dumela," I'd say. *Good day.*

"O kaai?" the object of my showing off would query. *How are you?*

"Ke teng. Wena okaai?" *I am well. How are you?*

"Ke teng."

"Sala sentle," I'd say, preparing to walk away. *Stay well.*

"Tsmaya sentle," my gracious responder would say. *Go well.*

While the Marikana massacre has, for now, defamiliarized the landscape I knew so intimately as a child, before too long dementia will likely have eroded that recently implanted memory and eased me back into the unspoiled idyll of a naïve child on an African farm. Like any childhood, though, mine was not without its own incursions of external eruptive forces, albeit of the not necessarily visible kind.

One week when I was about five years old, I was for some reason the only one of my family's then three siblings to accompany my mother to *die Jood* for grocery shopping. The minute my mother and I entered the store, Mrs. Katzenellenbogen abandoned the people she was serving at the black end of the counter—a "courtesy" she would have extended to any white customer—and came over to greet us. Or, rather, she greeted my mother. "And where is the pretty one today?" she asked.

I immediately understood that she was referring to my sister, Lana. While I do not subscribe to Freud's notion that childhood trauma necessarily becomes the central pivot of one's psychic makeup, I do admit that being marked as "not pretty" at the age of five could have had a dramatic impact on a child's self-image. However, I do not recall being scarred to the extent that I imagine my daughter or grand-daughter would be under similar circumstances. On our way home, my mother did raise the issue. "What a stupid woman," she said. "You are a very pretty girl." And that was all there was to it.

Today it seems unlikely to me that my mother's reassurance on its own would have been sufficient to erase a major psychic impact. Maybe it was because prettiness was not a value mentioned in our family other than as it related to landscapes, flowers, or clothes. The only mirror we had was hung at lipstick-application and shaving height in our one bathroom. Or maybe my father's love might have had something to do with my ego's apparent robustness. Whatever the reason, I did not cry or sulk or otherwise feel that my life had been ruined. If I felt put out about anything, it would more likely have been because, in the shop, my mother did not bring up the news that I had been transferred to grade two after only six months in grade one.

The real reason I survived the supposed psychic wound was probably far simpler: in an attempt to make up for her gaffe, Mrs. Katzenellenbogen had given me a lollipop.

It does not take forty-five years of marriage before one sees his or her partner in states of physical and/or psychic dishabillement that once seemed impossible in the rosy sepia of first love. The first instance of extreme discomposure happened for Peter and me—as I imagine it does for couples the world over—when our children were born. Not only does the birth itself entail the incursion of strangers into the most private parts of the woman's person *with her lover looking on*, but it also entails the insertion of an utterly dependent and exceedingly self-centered bundle of need into the fabric of their daily lives. And then there is the emotional depletion. Gone is the pre-baby niceness-in-the-face-of-difficulties that a couple in a harmonious relationship would usually have developed. *With baby looking on*, niceness gave way to eruptions of the id.

While our marriage did not lack the slinging of brutal "truths" during times of exceptional stress, Peter and I have always been able to reconnect at the core in times of crisis. I documented an example that took place during Marissa's birth in an article published in a South African women's magazine, *Fairlady*. After a first stage labor that went from sunrise to sunset on March 26, 1977,

my doctor judged the birth to be at least six hours off and went into town to see a play—he left his seat number with Peter. He had probably not even been ushered to his seat when I entered the transition stage—unfortunately with the full menu of classic manifestations, vomiting, shivering, a detached feeling, and the urge to push. From that time on, I could hear only Peter's voice. Through him, I relayed messages to the sister in attendance.

At 7 p.m. my waters broke. I was taken to the labour ward and my doctor's partner summoned. I'd never seen him before and rudely asked who he was. I refused to talk to him. Communication again took place through Peter, who at this stage also had to demonstrate the required breathing to me for each contraction.

For me, childbirth and parenting function as a schema of Peter's ability to keep loving me when matter gets the upper hand over mind. Most recently, he kept his cool during my theatre of the absurd performance after I underwent a surgical "readjustment" to non-cancer-related colon surgery that I had undergone two years earlier in 2012. Five days after the procedure, when the pain had already subsided and the incision in my nether parts was supposed to almost have healed, I was taking a shower when what I estimated to be a cup of blood suddenly gushed out. Shocked but calm, I cleaned myself up while trying to figure out how I was going to get Peter's attention. It was a Saturday morning and he was puttering in the garage about fifteen yards from where I was in the upstairs bathroom near the back door. Normally I would just yell out the window, but on that day I had no voice at all after a bout of the flu. I decided to summon him with a decorative dinner bell we keep on a kitchen counter. Stemming the blood with a wad of paper towel, I hunchbacked toward the bell, shuffled to the back door, and jangled the bell with my free hand. And so it came that a totally unsuspecting Peter walked out of the garage to see his naked wife framed in the door, one hand clutching a bloody wad of paper held to her crotch. Once we'd arrived at the emergency room, the surgeon replaced the stitches that had apparently come undone. Seven hours later Peter took me home and provided the TLC I needed until I was back to a less weak and pale version of my former self.

Since my microvascular disease diagnosis, I am only too aware that my mind is already buckling under the vagaries of matter. What worries me every day is the dishabillement of spirit that I visit upon my stalwart husband. While childbirth or a wound is temporary, my mental decline will be endless. As Peter and I already experience, my day-by-day drifts of attention are hard on both of us. I can only guess at the stress that the utterly dependent and exceedingly self-centered bundle of need that dementia will turn me into will provoke in him as my primary caretaker.

I do not doubt that Peter's heart is capacious enough to encompass the entire "rut of birth, love, pain, and death that crop[s] up unchanged for centuries." Our forty-eight-year relationship is testament to that. However, sometimes "nothing has time to gather meaning, and too many things are occurring for even a big heart to hold." When that time comes, our love must—will—be big enough to let go.

When we lived on our farm by Marikana, we were very poor. My mother would occasionally buy fabric from *die Jood* to make new dresses for herself, Lana, and me. For Christmas, my father's mother, Ouma Hansie, would buy a bolt of white cloth and give dress lengths to all the girl cousins so that their mothers could sew them matching dresses. My mother, ever creative, was always coming up with a collar or a sleeve or a flounce that none of the other cousins had. I would later have her eclecticism to thank for my own disregard for age-appropriateness when it comes to pattern or style.

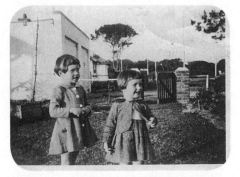

Gerda (age 4) and her sister Lana (age 3) in Cape Town, South Africa, just before the family moved to the family farm, 1953. Susanna made the dresses.

I acquired my first "bought" dress when Ouma Hansie's cousin from Rustenburg gave us some hand-me-downs. My first proper store-bought dress was occasioned by my confirmation during my standard nine or junior year of high school. It was navy blue with white piping, the colors making it suitable to be worn as a winter church dress at my boarding school after its debut at the farm church. Despite the practical constraints of its second purpose, it was a lovely dress that showed off my then adolescent-skinny figure. I wore it with a white pillbox hat for my confirmation. After its stint as my school church dress, it served a third term at university for my nice dress—this time without any headgear.

Once I had my first job, I finally was able to buy my own fabric—if rather sparingly, since my vacation salary had to pay for all my books plus school year needs beyond accommodation and food. During these student years, I sewed a number of dresses for class, work, and occasionally for dances. I emulated my mother's propensity to add a feature to those shown in the pattern—or subtract one, in the case of a shiny, long, pink body-fitting dance number, for which I omitted the left side seam to create a split up to my thigh. All the while I still incorporated hand-me-downs whenever they came my way.

After university, I experienced the luxury of now and then being able to buy a ready-made dress to supplement my still mostly home-made wardrobe. For my twenty-first birthday party, I acquired a macro-mini in a reflective silver fabric. I so treasured it that I stored it as a keepsake after minis had had their day. When Marissa was about five, I hauled it from its box and gave it to her. It hung down to her feet. She wore it until it had crept up her leg to mid-calf and loops of snagged silver threads hung down like tassels.

Dementia Field Notes

8-6-2013

I got dressed all the way to my shoes and earrings before I noticed that I had not put on a crucial piece of underwear.

8-17-2013

I've been having some clothing trouble. The other day I had to try about six times before I got my apron strings tied behind my back. And inside-out problems with underwear. Also some back-to-front issues with tops. When putting my pullover back on after having taken it off earlier in the day and leaving the arms inside out, I could not, as usual, get it back on.

———————

"We might not all read *Vogue*, but we still get dressed in the morning." So says Shira Tarrant and Marjorie Jolles in *Fashion Talks: Undressing the Power of Style*, a collection of essays that grew out of presentations at conferences of the National Women's Studies Association and the Cultural Studies Association.

Living in an increasingly visually mediated and commodified world means that having one's own style is compulsory. It is a core component of self-expression and self-realization. We need to look no further than our TVs for contemporary mythologies about identity, expression, and transformation as evidence of their cultural sway. Makeover shows of every type abound, whether the focus is on styling the corporeal body (*What Not to Wear*)…[or] the home (*Extreme Makeover: Home Edition*).

After raising the possibility of fashioning one's own style as "a core component of self-expression and self-realization," though, Tarrant and Jolles shatter the notion that one's self-presentation can ever be "true" to the wearer's own vision, since she does not have control over the "meaning" of her style of dress. "What fashion means depends on context, but also on whose interests it serves, what its audiences and practitioners bring to their engagement with it and how it protects and transforms social divisions."

Dementia Field Notes

6-11-2013

Since I started having trouble remembering which items go with what when I pick something to wear for the day, I have started now and then writing down the components of the outfit I wear.

That I survived the "not pretty" incident without much of a dent to my self-image does not mean that I am impervious to the shortcomings of my physical appearance. On the contrary. In addition to a number of small grievances I nurse, there have been three big ones: my tendency to gain weight easily has been a burr on my white school socks since, at the age of nine and in standard three—the equivalent of American fifth grade—I observed that I was chubby compared to Lana and my cousins. Since I wasn't fat enough (yet?) to be teased, I might not have paid my weight any heed had my mother not at this time become au courant with counting calories: probably imagining that she was done with babies after giving birth to four of us, she was on a post-childbearing makeover. She went on a strict diet. Since we did not have any bathroom scales, she would track her weight by dropping in at the doctor's office when we found ourselves in Marikana. Her primary feedback, though, was the notice she elicited from friends and family: compliments flowed from all directions. My mother was at pains to explain to her admirers that her diet was "scientific," i.e., based on a restricted calorie intake.

Without discussing it with anybody, I decided to reduce my calories, too: I stopped taking sandwiches to school for playtime and held out for dinner at home. My weight eventually stabilized at a body shape closer to that of my sister and cousins. I continued watching what I ate through elementary and high school and never again felt fat until I became an exchange student in the United States. During my year living with the Henning family in Breda, Iowa, I was no match for the temptations of American food, particularly that of my American mom, who was an excellent cook, and the pounds piled on. Toward the end of my year at Carroll High, and no doubt spurred on by the stress and excitement of the upcoming prom, I took to walking around the Carroll downtown rather than having school lunch. I dropped down to my pre-American weight.

After the births of each of my two children, I managed to return to a weight at which I felt good, albeit one higher than before I had my babies. Just before we emigrated from South Africa to the United States, the import of shifting our household across the Atlantic had worn me to the skinniest shape I had been since I planned my first pregnancy. Once in Utah, we lived in a hotel with a microwave and wash basin for a kitchen, and by necessity ate out for most of our main meals. Once we had found a house, our usual healthy eating often fell victim to the inexpensive possibilities of buying food that only had to be heated or, even worse, fast food. While my weight did not go completely overboard, it hit a higher peak than it ever had since my children were born.

Once I entered grad school in my forties, my figure went from bad to worse. Rather than the "freshman ten," I gained forty pounds, though over several years rather than all at once. There I became stuck until my mid-fifties. With the focus a steady job brings, I started exercising more and eating better, thereby losing the saddle of lard I had been packing for far too long. Since I have retired, it has become much easier to keep the creeping pounds at bay.

When I entered boarding school at age eleven and had daily access to a full-length mirror, my sparse allotment of thin brown hair became a second bugbear. In my last year of high school I caught the anxiety about the upcoming Matric dance. Since there was a girl in my wing who did hair, I felt mature—and even pretty—with my hair done up. The next year, as an exchange student back in high school, I was astonished at how much effort my peers put into their hair. American high school was a breeze after the South African Matric, so I, too, took more time with my hair and washed it more frequently than the once-a-week shampoo encouraged at boarding school. That, together with my first regular access to a blow dryer, helped separate the fine strands into a fullness that at least ensured my scalp would not shine through. In my fifties when I went to much shorter hair, I happily tossed out the hair dryer. Today my hair is even shorter, a crew cut in fact. It is almost white, though a little bit of gray still lurks at the back of my head. Like my Kalahari grandmother, I had started sprouting gray strands in my twenties.

My maternal Ouma Truia's hair had been a wonder that fascinated me as a child. When I was in elementary school and she in her fifties, it was already all white. She wore it in a bun. During our month-long yearly visits, she let it loose of an evening so I could brush it. It was soft and shiny and smelled of Lifebuoy soap and malva pudding. Once a week, she invited me to the back *stoep* to help her wash it in an enamel basin with black poxes where the white had chipped off. Since the farmhouse's water was cranked from a well that ran dry during droughts and the buckets had to be carried seventy yards to the kitchen, water was used sparingly. After the first wash, I would carry the sloshing basin to the pepper tree and slowly empty it around the trunk. For the final rinse, Ouma would let me fetch clean water from the kitchen where the day's two buckets were each covered with a muslin cloth. Taking care not to spill one drop, I would measure five cups into a magnum-sized enamel jug enhanced with a blue, pink, yellow, and green flower pattern and bear it to the *stoep* to dribble over Ouma's hair while she worked out the last bit of soap. The remaining water was still clean enough for washing my own hands and feet.

My nostalgia about Ouma Truia's hair meant that my early graying never bothered me. Through my thirties and forties, I rather liked the white strips that started outlining my ears, and I made no attempt to hide them. Midway through graduate school when I started thinking about job prospects, though—upon the advice of friends my age who occupied lofty positions on their own career ladders—I took to coloring the white strips medium brown to match the yet un-grayed hair on the rest of my head. Those white parts did not take kindly to the makeover: they did not take color well and the roots also grew out very rapidly. I had to apply color every two weeks not to feel unkempt. And so I battled on through two different jobs in the corporate world over a period of seven years.

A few years into my University of Utah position in Gender Studies I decided that coming out as a gray-haired sage in an environment where diversity of all stripes was supported and encouraged would be the sensible thing to do. Accordingly, I cut my hair very short and grew out the roots. Even I was surprised at how different I looked—during the years of coloring, my hair had turned as white as my Ouma's. For the first time in my life, my hair was a trigger for more compliments than I had ever had before about any physical feature.

From my forties onward, when my inheritance of the family jowls had become evident as a result of my PhD program weight gain, the pocket of fat dangling below my chin became a third bête noir on my list of gene-determined attributes I would rather be without. I knew from family examples that my neck would eventually turn into whole cascades of fat-filled folds. Telling only my family and closest friends, I succumbed to liposuction. I have never spent a ridiculous sum of money on a more worthwhile shallow activity. I liked my face in the mirror so much better—for almost two decades. At the time of my liposuction, my surgeon had said that I would need "a tightening up" when I was older. He was right. However, now that I am in my sixties, I have become resigned to settling for that much-fêted and, in my opinion, greatly overrated "inner beauty." However, I am not yet beyond distracting people from the havoc time is playing with my features by gearing my clothes to the age I *feel* rather than look. As Maya Angelou, the famed poet whose unretouched magnificence reaped her as one of *Glamour*'s 2009 Women of the Year, puts it, "The most important thing I can tell you about aging is this: If you really feel that you want to have an off-the-shoulder blouse and some big beads and thong sandals and a dirndl skirt and a magnolia in your hair, do it. Even if you're wrinkled."

Dementia Field Notes

3-2-2014

I am trying to change from my winter to my spring wardrobe. I have been working on this for several days, but just can't seem to get my closet organized. When I try to arrange my clothes in the same logical order as I have always done—hanging the major components of an outfit side-by-side—it does not seem to work anymore because there are a few tops and long T-shirts I wear under short tops that I mix and match in different ways for different outfits. In the olden days it didn't matter, because I could remember the different combinations. I have lately found that I get very confused if I start mixing outfits around: I forget some possibilities—even my favorites—for weeks on end. So the decision I had to make was: outfits together or pants, shirts, skirts, etc. grouped together "each according to their kind" like the animals in Noah's ark. I have tried working on it today, but as I tried to implement the "each according to their kind" option, I knew that on a daily basis I would never be able to remember what to put together with what to create the mixes I really love. I had earlier written down some winter outfits in my journal to remember them, but that seems impossibly complicated to do for all my clothes.

3-7-2014

I had an idea of how the "each according to their kind" clothing arrangement could work: I'm going to take my time, put together all the various outfits I can think of, and take photos. So I have launched the huge project of setting out each outfit on the bed and taking pictures. Peter took me to Walmart to get a mini-photo album to keep the photos together so I could easily consult them. I've been taking photos for days now and have printed the daily batches as I go along. This morning I got the last of the photos taken and printed and looked forward to putting the clothes guide together. However, the photos I had printed in daily batches were utterly lost. I could not find them anywhere in the house. So I printed them again, and now finally have my mnemonic device ready for use.

———

One of my favorite pieces of jewelry is a memento mori ("remember that you will die") pendant that I wear on a chain together with a same-length string of pearls. The pendant, made by American designer Betsey Johnson—known for her over-the-top and embellished work and her performance of a cartwheel at her fashion shows—is a 5 inch long by 1½ inch wide white-enameled and bejeweled skeleton that declares itself as female with a red-yellow-orange fringy skirt and a hat made out of multicolored enameled fruit and rhinestones in primary colors. Her heart is represented with a glittering costume ruby fixed to the left of her sternum so that it sits lightly atop one of her ribs.

The other day when I was wearing the pendant, the skeleton's sternum and heart clicked out of the clasps that attach them to the rest of her. Fortunately, jewelry is among the wide variety of items that Peter alters and repairs for me. I put the broken-hearted skeleton on Peter's red toolbox in his study, meaning to ask him to fix it, but then forgot. The next morning, I found my skeleton-girl on the kitchen counter, still in two parts, and neatly laid out in a paper coffin that Peter had made for her—complete with a headstone enjoining her to RIP. After we had hooted about his joke, he fixed her heart, as he always does mine.

In the "Ask a Woman" column on the website Dappered—"for guys who value and feel most comfortable in a classic, sharp, tailored style...but also value having a real savings account and retirement plan"—Beth writes that "each of us engages with fashion and style whether we want to or not." Beth goes on:

> [Do] men dress for women, and women dress for...other women? [Why, then] do women wear [clothes] that...men say they dislike? At its worst, women dress to one-up other women because we are socialized to compete with each other for attention and positive reinforcement in a way that men are not...Our motivations [are not necessarily] to be sexi*er,*

thinn*er*, prett*ier* [than our friends], but mostly less nefarious: we just really care about being perceived by other women as well-dressed and attractive.

I wear clothing that I find beautiful and fun and elegant, hoping that some of those qualities will rub off on me while I wear those pieces.

Other fashionistas have their say:

Lady Gaga: I'm just trying to change the world, one sequin at a time.

Alexander the Great: A tomb now suffices him for whom the adornment of an entire world was not sufficient.

Aliya, holding the two halves of a broken plastic whiffle ball to her chest: I have boo-boos. (After a moment's contemplation.) I don't actually have boo-boos—yet. I will get them when I grow up.

Dementia Field Notes, 7-26-2014: The other day I put my bra on over my pajama T-shirt.

The Church of Jesus Christ of Latter Day Saints: "Modesty is an attitude of propriety and decency in dress, grooming, language, and behavior. If we are modest, we do not draw undue attention to ourselves. Instead, we seek to 'glorify God in [our] body, and in [our] spirit' (1 Corinthians 6:20; see also 1 Corinthians 6:19)…If we are unsure about whether our dress or grooming is modest, we should ask ourselves, 'Would I feel comfortable with my appearance if I were in the Lord's presence?'"

Ouma Truia: My little lamb, do you know someone who can give you some boy clothes to mail to me? The Hotnots who came here to help with the fence repairs are still here and they have a boy—I reckon he's about six or seven—who is wearing a dress. I told his mother to put pants on him, but they don't have any. He has nothing on under the dress, not even girl bloomers. I just cannot behold this anymore. Deuteronomy says that if a man wears a woman's clothes it is an abomination to the Lord God. We can't have this thing going on at the farm any more.

Dementia Field Notes

9-23-2013

Last week I was shopping in Nordstrom and decided to try on a gorgeous gray-with-a-lilac-cast sweater. Since Peter was about to pick me up, I thought I would just try it on in front of one of the store mirrors rather than go into a dressing room. I found a mirror, put all my stuff down, and when I next looked at myself in the mirror with proper awareness, I saw that I had taken off my shirtdress and was standing there in my underwear from the waist up. I quickly put my shirtdress on again and then tried the sweater over it, as I had originally intended. I was shaken. I don't think anyone noticed. I could have been arrested for indecent exposure!

In the first photo ever taken of my mother, she must have been about three years old. She and her brother Pieter are both sitting on the lap of her maternal grandfather, a man with a Walt Whitman as old man full white beard and blue eyes that stare sorrowfully from deep, dark sockets. Two-year-old Pieter, whose hair is blond in the photo, has a facial structure exactly the same as his grandfather's. In contrast with these two souls who appear as if they will not sojourn long in this world, Susanna's full face and sparkly dark eyes look flushed with vitality. She wears a simple white dress, white socks, and black shoes. Her shoulder-length, almost-black hair is drawn back from her forehead in a big, silky, chocolate-box bow, a vanity uncharacteristic of her family's food-scarce, bookless, and toyless existence.

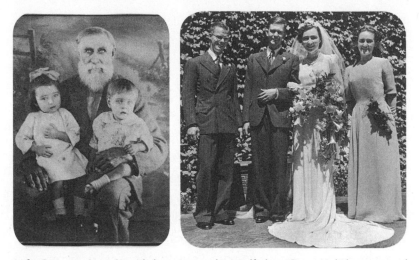

Left, Susanna (age 3) with her maternal grandfather, Oupa Holtzhauzen, and younger brother Pieter Myburgh, approximately 1927. Right, Boshoff and Susanna get married, Cape Town, South Africa, 1948. Susanna made her own wedding dress and bouquet.

Whether she had inherited the parental sensibility that had added the ribbon to her outfit or been inspired by the feeling of being special in her family by her only-girl status, Susanna always regarded a stylish manner of dress as her due. From her "courting" portraits with my father to her exquisite long lace wedding dress and bridal bouquet spilling tendrils all the way to her knees— both of which she made herself—through to her mid-seventies, she maintained a personal style that was a notch above the ordinary. During her final six or seven years, however, her hair (though clean) always looked somewhat unkempt and she mostly wore—or was dressed in—the South African equivalent of the "sexy crystal bling velour sweat suit with drawstring pants for easy toileting" that gave me the creeps when it popped up during an internet search for exercise wear. On the whole, she did not seem to be bothered by her appearance—at least during my visits.

After my mother had become considerably impaired, my direct communication with her took place only by phone. Now and then she would say that "she had nothing to wear." In the same vein, my sister-in-law June reported Susanna's lament that she did not have "enough shiny things," since "they" had stolen everything. While it is possible that a member of the staff or one of Susanna's care center neighbors, similarly robbed of rationality, had pilfered them, it is more likely that "they" were the same people who at the time were "broadcasting from the wall of my bedroom."

No matter the reason behind Susanna's sartorial deficit, I asked June to buy her some costume jewelry on my behalf—mailing parcels to South Africa often resulted in "them" stealing the contents before the item had been delivered. Saint June procured a "brooch with many diamonds": a circular confection that consists of silver tendrils of filigree tastefully finished in a matte style and adorned with sky-blue confetti of rhinestones. Now, after her death, I frequently pin it on, not only in remembrance of my mother, but also because it is the kind of over-the-top accessory I sometimes go for.

On August 19, 2013—a day so warm that the notion of fall seemed unimaginable—I took the bus downtown to City Creek Center. It is adjacent to the Mormon Church's world headquarters at Temple Square, spans three blocks in the heart of downtown, and incorporates upscale stores as well as residential buildings. A river runs through it, albeit a simulated one. It boasts two waterfalls, three fountains, and a number of trout pools. The stores are connected by foliage-lined walkways and a skyway across Main Street. A retractable roof opens up to the springtide; in summer and winter, it unfurls into a glass-paneled cathedral ceiling that alternately cocoons air-conditioned coolness or furnace-rendered warmth.

My shopping expedition that day to City Creek Center was not geared toward gawking at its pleasing architectural features or supporting the local economy, other than maybe through the purchase of a cup of coffee. My hope was rather to attain a state of relaxed mindfulness that had eluded me for several weeks of being bogged in a malaise bordering on depression.

The endorphin-upping exercise I'd had in mind for my mall outing combined three of my usually successful stimuli: (1) do something you're scared of, in this case take the bus, a formerly simple task I now dreaded after lately botching it once or twice, (2) engage in a physical activity you like (walk), and (3) stimulate the senses you frequently override with too much thinking (imbibe the murmur of the brook and redolence of wet rocks and plants; ingest the colors and compositions of the store displays).

On this Monday afternoon, however, no amount of nature or commerce succeeded in penetrating my slump. While I traversed the walkways, neither fish ponds nor fountains set my thoughts in free flow; inside the stores, neither fashions nor fads took me to a place beyond words. Unless I were willing to admit defeat and catch the bus home, I would have to exert tougher pressure on those ornery anodyne dispensers. So I devised a plan B: Search for a more definite goal. Stage an opportunity for rapid gratification. Go on a specific quest rather than allowing "God's water to flow across God's acre," as an Afrikaans expression has it.

The goal I settled on was to find something "grown-up" to wear in the mall's anchor stores, Nordstrom and Macy's. Something other than the riotously colorful clothing rainbowing my closet. My task did not include having to buy anything. I merely had to locate an object outside the range of my usual eccentric taste, an outfit in which I could blend in a room of smartly dressed people and that I would love to own. For the next two hours, I would be free from price constraints. Also, I would ignore dry-clean-only considerations or such practicalities as whether my life in Utah involved many rooms of smartly dressed people.

An hour or so into my quest, nothing had jumped out at me. Our state's designer market, at least as interpreted by Nordstrom, appeared to be geared toward classical elegance in the manner of, say, Isabella Rossellini instead of creative dressers like Paloma Picasso.

In Nordstrom, the most promising of my two options, my pace petered into a desultory amble when I finally laid my eyes on an item I desired: a Marc by Marc Jacobs dress in "persian purple," with a design of saucer-sized red and white tulips coupled with lili-aceous leaves in the same colors.

A spurt of endorphins gave my mood a boost. With a lift in my step, I crossed the sky bridge to try my luck at Macy's as well. Half an hour later, I'd had no luck in the designer or any other clothing section, but I was determined to not let go of the perk the Persian purple dress had given me. I decided to have a quick look at the jewelry downstairs on my way out. My bus home was due soon.

Macy's designer section is on the second floor. Even though I was in a hurry, I glanced about for stairs rather than opting for the escalator—I had made a habit of expending energy as part of my daily routine rather than counting on going to the gym, which I skipped at every excuse. Amid the many red exit signs on the floor, I spotted a green one at the shoe section. I wandered over, opened the door, and entered the stairwell. Once I reached the ground floor, I saw that I had arrived at a street door rather than one I had expected would let me directly back into the store. Uttering an expletive, I pushed the release bar. It did not budge. I tried a few more times, pushing harder with my hands, and then resorted to a thrust with my hip. All in vain.

I had by now wasted the time I'd had left for the jewelry, so I took the stairs back up to reenter the store by the door through which I had landed in the stairwell. Back at the second-floor landing, my annoyance about missing out on the jewelry changed to panic: there was no door handle. The door through which I had exited was a fire door—once you were in the stairwell you could not go back in.

This place has only three exits, sir: Madness, and Death.

I ran up the stairs to the third floor, just in case that door were different. It was not. I went down again to the landing where I had earlier entered the stairwell and sat down on the steps. I noticed how hot it was. Sweat was beading on my forehead and starting to drip through my eyebrows. The exit into which I had bumbled was apparently in an outside corner of the store and both of the outside walls must have baked in the sun all day.

I felt dehydrated, craved water. I decided to put my bodily discomforts from my mind. I needed every bit of thinking energy to figure my way out. A serenity came over me. I stepped through my options:

1. Bang on the door and shout.

    Failure. The door is solid metal and the dull sound from my banging fists does not carry.

2. Lie down on the floor to shout through the quarter-inch crack where the door meets the floor.

    Con, floor covered in oily-looking grime. Worse, if someone suddenly opened the door, it would smash into my face. Too dangerous to try.

3. Phone mall security.

Not possible—I don't have a smart phone (too complex to operate with my memory) to Google the number.

4. Call Peter.

Con, one of my afternoon's goals was to spare him the chauffeuring that he has been doing since I gave up driving. Try to avoid this one.

5. Marissa and Adam?

M takes after me and doesn't lightly answer her cell phone unless she is away from Dante; A usually answers. Possibility.

6. Newton or Cheryl?

Usually answer, but live half-hour away.

7. 911?

Seems overly dramatic.

I opted for calling Peter. "I'm really in trouble," I said. I told him the story. His response was that he was going to jump in the car and come let me out. I suggested that he instead call the Macy's office and ask that security rescue me. He ostensibly agreed. I described my location, he phoned, and about five minutes later I received a call from a security guard. He was on his way.

By the time the guard—a young man named Junior who had the shape of a bodybuilder—found me, I had been in the stairwell for about twenty minutes. I felt light-headed from the heat and asked for water. I also asked to see the store manager. Junior delivered me to the management office. While I waited for the manager, an apparently second-in-charge administrator, Todd, offered me lots of water and a half-hearted apology. By the time I'd had two bottles of water Peter walked in. He was very concerned and hugged me several times to make sure I was okay. The store manager, Wendy, showed up, demonstrating solicitude and offering apologies with an HR workshop-honed competence. She sent Todd and Junior to investigate how I got stuck behind an emergency door to the street that was supposed to remain open at all times and listened to my concerns.

When the investigators returned, their first news was apologetic. Someone had neglected to arm the door, which would have turned the red light red and set off an alarm when I used it. Their next words, though not an accusation, underhandedly turned the blame back on me. There was a warning on the door, they said, informing customers not to use it and stating that an alarm would go off if the door were opened. I could not argue that. I had seen those warnings many times before. Peter and I later checked that it had indeed been in place. In my hurry to see the jewelry, though, I had not noticed it at all.

I could forgive myself my failure to read the notice. When I had looked for an exit, the large green LED sign above the door had trumped the small black letters of the notice in vying for my attention. The next part of Todd's account, however, floored me. The street door had not been locked, he said, "you just have to push a bit hard."

Though Peter later told me that he thought their story was a butt-covering ploy, I right away believed it possible that I had not pushed the door hard enough or in the right place. Hadn't I experienced failures to take note of relevant sensory information for months? Weren't my Dementia Field Notes blotted with accounts of me not noticing that the toilet lid was closed until I had peed all over it? Or needed Peter's help to find my radio, which was in its usual place on the kitchen windowsill? I have learned the truth of the idea that one sees with your brain, not your eyes.

As is often the case in situations where different observers have different accounts, the matter of whether the door had actually been secured—against homeless wanderers, entering through the store, looking for shelter?—with a pin that could be pulled out in an emergency by Macy's cognoscenti (as Peter suspected) or whether it had been just a bit hard to open (as the employees reported and I feared) was never resolved.

That night I called my friend Kirstin to bewail the ignominy of having been swallowed whole by a stairwell.

"You poor thing," she said. "You are trapped in a metaphor."

My good laugh, coming after the adrenalin-doling drama of the Macy's lockup, distracted me from my deep blue blahs for a few hours into the night. The fog, which murked my mood again the next morning, only lifted after I gave in and visited my doctor, who adjusted my medication.

For my birthday a month later, Kirstin gave me a Macy's gift certificate with a drawing on the envelope of me in a locked stairwell. I was not alone. I was companionably surrounded by her and her family. My mind swerved. The vehicle of the metaphor was no longer a barren trap, but had metamorphosed into a congenial cocoon, like a station wagon traveling across the country with a family belting out road trip songs all along the way.

With the gift card I bought myself a pair of jeans the color of crushed blueberries. They have skinny legs and an overall fit snugger than what most Utah women my age who aspire to dress well would wear in public. Nothing grown-up about them.

I am increasingly aware that my vanity about my clothing style is something that I will probably have to give up when I can no longer get dressed or—horrors!—even select an outfit without help. That moment is much on my mind every time I stare at my closet trying to construct what clothes and jewelry I had combined before. I'm afraid my projects of writing down and/or photographing my outfits have, for the moment, come to an end. It takes me so long to write and just take care of myself that I have not been able to keep up my mnemonic system. That I cannot even manage that at the moment forces me to ask, "Once I need even more help to live in the world than I do now, would it be reasonable to expect someone else to pursue my fashion quirks on behalf of a no-longer-existing Gerda-self?" Isn't letting go of the things of the world part of the transformation I must undergo as I enter zombiehood? How can I put the burden of replicating an aesthetic that I have cultivated over the years—and which, moreover, I regularly adapt to my constantly changing sense of self—on someone already spending their lumpen time on me?

Would one of my family members like the task of dolling up a Senior Citizen Barbie?

Kanye doesn't seem to care much about how he dresses other than that his clothes are not to hamper his wildly athletic activities in any way. Dante, however, even though he is only three, is showing a promising exactitude about doing everything according to the rules he has figured out for himself. Shoes are his specialty. Even when he could barely walk, he would dutifully match abandoned shoes with their owners and repeat "Tjoo, tjoo," until the laggard had put them back on. Most promising, though, is his *Sex and the City*–style adoration of his red Elmo slip-ons.

Of the three grandkids, Aliya is so far showing the most interest in developing her own Mardi Gras style of dress. When she was only two, she used to sneak her mom's bra to wear under her dress whenever she had the chance. When she was almost three and Christmas rolled around, I came upon the tiniest, flattest starter bra I had ever seen, on sale for a dollar. I checked with Newton and Cheryl and they said it was okay to buy it: I bought the only two left, one pink, the other dove-gray.

Not able to let go of a good thing when it gets me ouma points, this past Christmas I bought her two new bras: a yellow one with pink binding and straps and a purple one with touches of green. Aliya, though, has moved on.

Like me, my granddaughter focuses her attention now on what immediately strikes the eye. She specializes in unusual clothing and accessories: nonmatching socks, even nonmatching shoes, tights of every stripe, hair styles that involve sparkly clips and bows and flower finishes—when I do her hair we go for fresh flowers—and glittery skirts that go over dresses, tights, her ballet costume, her winter coat, a pair of jeans, and so on. I believe I have found a willing receiver for my clothing Olympics. For now, we are still running side-by-side in the passing zone. Far be it from me, while I am still rational, to issue an edict that hapless family members attend Doña Quixote's toilette "for a considerable portion of each day" in order to deck her out in a royal robe and diadem. Unless it gives him or her pleasure.

Until, as will eventually happen for all of us, personal pleasure comes to an end.

Ecclesiastes 3:19: For that which befalleth the sons of men befalleth beasts; even one thing befalleth them: as the one dieth, so dieth the other; yea, they have all one breath; so that a man hath no preeminence above a beast: for all is vanity.

Mrs. Katzenellenbogen: And where is the pretty one today?

Doña Quixote: I have nothing to wear.

Jane Austen: Vanity working on a weak head produces every sort of mischief.

According to a fable alive among Greek seamen today, a solitary mermaid would grasp a ship's prow during a storm and ask the captain, "Is Megalexandros alive?" The person the mermaid is enquiring about is Alexander the Great, of course. Given the historical datum that the Greek general died over two thousand years ago, it is not surprising that the uninitiated might come back with the literal truth, "No." Upon hearing this answer, the mermaid would turn into a raging Gorgon with a corona of writhing snakes and a visage so dreadful that her beholder, together with all other hands on board, would turn to stone. The unintended ballast would cause the ship to sink to the bottom of the ocean.

Those who know better would not dare give a response other than "He is alive and well and rules the world!" Gentled by the correct answer, the mermaid would vanish and the storm dissipate, leaving "only mild and lulling airs to refresh the souls of men."

Chapter Eight

The Exit That Dare Not Say Its Name

This place has only three exits, sir: Madness, and Death.
—René Daumal

WHEN OUR FAMILY FIRST arrived in Utah in August 1984 we lived in a cheap furnished motel with a kitchenette. Our "suite" opened onto a piece of property that has since been developed into a commercial building, but at the time was a field covered in switch-grass and weeds where our children, seven-year-old Marissa and four-year-old Newton, spent the month of August catching Mormon crickets. As soon as Peter got home from work, we would meet a real estate agent and go house hunting. We had decided to sink all of the money we were able to bring from South Africa—the amount was restricted, we had been allowed less than half of our life earnings until then—into a house. It was barely enough for the down payment. Just before the start of school, we found a neglected but spacious house (to accommodate all the visitors from South Africa we were hoping for) in the Wasatch foothills, in a suburb about half an hour south of the city center. Our street was called· Supernal Way.

Despite the fact that our furniture and other household goods were still en route, we moved in right away so the children could start school at Cottonwood Elementary. Before we had time to purchase even a few basic household items, though, the neighbors discovered our minimalist living status. Not surprisingly, our intention to "camp out" in our house struck them as refugee-like— we were, after all, from Africa! By day's end, our kindly new acquaintances had loaned us sleeping bags, a standing lamp for the living room, a coffee table, and a few other items. After carrying a picnic table from the deck into the kitchen, buying a microwave, and stocking up on paper plates, we were ready to start our life in America—far better equipped than the pioneers who crossed the prairie with handcarts about whom our kids would soon start learning in school.

Our camp-out, which we had not expected to go on for more than a few weeks, stretched into months—the shipping container bearing our material possessions from South Africa had mistakenly been dispatched on a European grand tour. It finally caught up with us just before Thanksgiving. When we got word that "our medium-sized dry goods" had finally arrived on American soil, we were ecstatic. As soon as our furniture was delivered and lugged to the assigned places, we tackled the most crucial boxes. The familiar objects we unearthed took on the luster of long-lost treasure. Overnight, they turned our encampment into home.

Our children, too, were "out of their skins," as we say in Afrikaans, about at last being surrounded with their familiar bedroom furniture, books, clothes, and toys. An unexpected consequence, though, was that they finally internalized the fact that our move to the United States was permanent. It sank in that their cousins and friends and oumas, with whom they had played amid the same furniture and with the same toys, would be absent from their daily lives for a long time. They would not be with them for birthdays, Christmases, or sleepovers. Newton went to bed night after night clutching a piece of Lego and crying, "I just want to play with Craig," his over-the-fence neighbor from Parktown North. Marissa, being older and more likely to stew out emotions in her head before talking, did not show her distress with the same abandonment. Sometime before Christmas, the gears that had been churning in her brain produced a question of the kind no parent likes to answer: "Who will look after me and Newton if you and Daddy die, not when you're very old and we are grown up, but now?"

Fortunately, her question came out when we were having dinner. Newton, who had turned five the first week in November, joined his sister with a questioning look. In as matter-of-fact a tone as we could muster, and with frequent mutual interruptions and rephrasings, Peter and I reminded them that their godparents, my sister Lana and her husband, Buzz, would take care of them if we died, though we would probably not die for a long, long time. We explained that even though we were *here* and Tannie Lana and Uncle Buzz over *there*, they would come and get them and take them back to South Africa, where all their aunts and uncles as well as their two grandmothers, Ouma Raaitjie and Ouma Susan, would help look after them. With more brio than we felt, we invoked their same-age cousins, Lana and Buzz's children John and Julia, and told them they would live together and be able to play every day.

"I know," Marissa said, her look indicating that our answers had been too elementary.

"When we live with Tannie Lana," Newton whooped, "she can take me to Craig's house and I can play with him."

Marissa worried on. "But they don't know where we live."

I reminded her that we had called her godparents some weeks earlier and that we gave them our address and phone number. Peter, reading another need in her question, wrote the information for making an international call on a card and taped it to the wall by the phone. All the while Newton steered his one-track train to the next station. "Or sometimes Craig can come to their house and we can play in the treehouse."

"Who will make us food and take us to school before they get here?" Marissa wanted to know.

Finally figuring out that we had now gotten to what was probably the proximate source of her anxiety, Peter and I again rehearsed the arrangement about which we had told the children some weeks earlier: the families of their new school friends, Hilary who lived just up the road and Nathan who lived near the school, would take care of them if Peter and I were unable to do so. With a guilty glance at each other, Peter and I wordlessly acknowledged that what we had had in mind at the time we spoke to our new friends were the smaller vicissitudes of life, such as snowstorms or car breakdowns.

We had gotten to know these couples in the quick way people sometimes bond with the parents of their children's best friends. What loomed rather large in our new friendships was the fact that none of us belonged to the Mormon church. While Peter and I arrived in Salt Lake City knowing it was the headquarters of the Church of Jesus Christ of Latter-Day Saints (LDS), we were oblivious to how much that circumstance affects ordinary life in Utah. One of the first things people ask new neighbors is what ward, or local congregation, you belong to. People are friendly enough when you confess that you're not a member of the church. However, the chances of forming true friendships are very slim, since the lives of one's Mormon neighbors are almost entirely consumed by their church. Even ordinary activities like pick-up basketball games or block parties are facilitated by the church. Besides, the church keeps its members extremely busy—church responsibilities eat up most of the time that people in non-Mormon environments would use to develop close friendships.

Another obstacle toward friendships among Mormons and non-Mormons is that unless you are on the local ward's remarkably efficient phone chain, major local events go by without you knowing about them. For example, when the adult daughter of our neighbors across the road was dying at their home, I had—like many other neighbors—often walked over with cookies or another small treat for the daughter and once or twice stayed with her when her grief-stricken and overworked mother went out for an errand, but I only heard about her death after the funeral.

As the social sphere of our new neighborhood slowly dawned on us, Peter and I were delighted that we had met potential "real" friends in the parents of our children's friends. We all got to know each other well in a short time. Well enough that I told both the Taylors and the Shands the tale of a traumatic event that befell us during our second week in our new house. Marissa's asthma flared up in a severe attack, and we had had to rush her to the hospital.

We had been aware of the seriousness of Marissa's asthma already in South Africa, where she had more than once been hospitalized after a very sudden escalation of her illness during a cold. Though her asthma had been well controlled for the last year or two in South Africa, we were always concerned and on the alert when she contracted any upper-respiratory infection—no less so in a new country where we had not yet even found a doctor. When, on an evening two weeks into our occupation of our new house, Marissa's chest became very tight and her breathing strained, we knew it was time to get medical help fast. We knew that we had a long night ahead. Casting myself on the mercy of the neighbors—who also happened to be non-Mormon—who had loaned us the lamp and the coffee table and with whose boys Newton had subsequently played a few times, I unceremoniously appeared at their doorstep with Newton, already in his pajamas, and asked if he could sleep over. Their immediate grasp of our situation and open-armed welcome brought tears to my eyes. At the emergency room, Marissa was found to be very ill and she was admitted to the hospital, where she stayed for three days, during which Peter or I hardly ever left her side. Watching over her pale, quiet form, I thought about death in the midst of our new life. "If she dies now," my heart cried, "there will be no one who knows her at her funeral except us."

Eventually, the what-if-Mamma-and-Daddy-died cloud seemed to have cleared. We moved on to thinking about another major event that would make our house on Supernal Way an even more home-like space: the arrival of our two large, furry, black dogs that we had left in South Africa. In those days, pets could only be brought into the United States legally after a three-week quarantine in American-government-licensed kennels in their home country, at the end of which they had to pass a health test. We'd gotten word from my brother Carel that they had been declared healthy and that he would be putting them on the plane right away.

The next day, we all went to the airport to pick up Kwaaitjie, a Standard Poodle, and Liewe Heks, a Bouvier des Flandres. The airport had a special building some distance away from the terminals where we would be reunited with our dogs. When an attendant handed them over to us, they just about flattened us in their joy to see us.

Once we had brought the dogs home, it felt as if another layer of normal had been gentled over our alien shoulders. However, oblivious of what their quarantine and plane tickets had cost us, our dogs soon repaid our efforts to make Americans of them by acting as if they had been raised by wolves: they viciously attacked a cat that had ventured into our backyard.

I first learned about our animals' transgression one morning when Newton shouted, in Afrikaans, from the back lawn, "Ek het 'n halwe dooie kat gekry," which translates to "I found half a dead cat." As in English, the sentence has a sibling that is very similar in grammar but has a very different meaning: "I found a half-dead cat." Given my five-year-old's grasp of his mother tongue, which he now heard only in his home, I could not be sure which of these meanings he'd had in mind. "Not half a dead cat, Newton!" I shouted as I sprinted down the stairs to see the extent of the injuries for myself. However, what Newton carried toward me by its tail confirmed that there had been nothing amiss with my son's grammar.

That evening when Peter got home, he and I scoured the backyard for other parts of the cat, but found none. Our whole family then walked door to door along our street, Peter and I hoping that our prepared apology and pleas for the lives of our children's furry, black canine security blankets would sway the bereaved pet owner to resist calling whatever animal police force Utah might have. Despite our broadcasting of the horrible news around the neighborhood, no one claimed the remains of the cat. Our stations of the cross completed, we locked the dogs up in the house and buried the unfortunate animal's remains in the large unlandscaped hillside portion of our backyard. We stood around the grave talking about how the cat's molecules would mix with the soil and feed the trees and shrubs we were going to plant and that its atoms might become part of a tree trunk or a leaf or a flower. After the funeral, the children collected rocks and built a marker of stones that, in addition to its function as a memorial, would prevent the perpetrators' return to the scene for the commission of even more unspeakable acts on the victim's remains.

That night, after Peter and I had read the kids their bedtime story and just as I was ready to kick back in my easy chair, Newton padded into the room clad in his pajamas. Not wanting to miss out should her brother's extension of his bedtime reap any privileges, Marissa slunk into the living room as well. Newton, however, was not trying to weasel a sip of juice or a piece of cheese out of us. Instead, he had an urgent question. "Can someone be dead if they're not ripped in half?"

While it did not take parental genius to figure out that our son's question had been triggered by the day's grisly event, it took Newton's next question for us to realize that we had arrived back at the what-if-Mamma-and-Daddy-die conundrum: "Who will help us dig the holes when you and Daddy are dead?" After another round of assurances that plenty of adults would be available to help them in the very, very, very unlikely event of our simultaneous deaths, Peter and I went back to Newton's earlier question about how one knows someone is dead. Since I had read in a magazine that one should not compare death to sleep when discussing it with young children since that might make them afraid of bedtime, I launched into an explanation of how your heart stops beating when you die. We then felt each other's pulses at the wrist and neck, after which Peter worked every ticklish spot he could think of on each of our offspring. Soon we were all laughing and wrestling on the carpet. In the end Newton's question got him and Marissa not only a full-family snuggle fest, but also a glass of milk and a cookie to take away the taste of unpalatable information from their *parents'* mouths.

Once the kids were back in bed, Peter poured us each a glass of wine. We sank into our couch holding hands and asking ourselves whether our quest for better opportunities balanced out our children's loss of innocence.

Like all what-ifs, this one has no answer.

*   *   *

At the close of 2010, while I was absorbing the implications of my dementia prognosis, a conceptual art piece by Damien Hirst was completing its three-year residence at the Metropolitan Museum of Modern Art. It consisted of a tiger shark floating in twenty-three tons of formaldehyde contained in a steel-and-glass vitrine. On sunny days, light from the bank of windows behind it brought out the sky-blue cast of the embalming fluid. Daylight brought out the dark stripes down the shark's body that resemble a tiger's pattern. At the head end of the rectangular tank, the animal's wide open mouth drew your eye through a fortress of jagged teeth into the black hole of its gullet. After dusk, the window reflected the tank back at you, doubling the shark into parentheses that seemed to embrace life and death simultaneously.

Hirst titled the work *The Physical Impossibility of Death in the Mind of Someone Living*, "a statement that [he] had used to describe the idea of death to [himself]" while writing his student thesis on hyperreality during the late 1980s. He "liked its poetic clumsiness because of the way it expressed, 'something that wasn't there, or was there.' "

Hirst's opportunity to transform the idea in his thesis into a sculpture came in 1989 when British advertising magnate and contemporary art collector Charles Saatchi commissioned him to create a conceptual piece of his choice for the businessman's eponymous gallery. The artist engaged an Australian fisherman to capture a tiger shark "big enough to eat you." The fisherman obliged with a fish of which the length, in today's conceptual currency, would add up to the tallest and shortest NBA players of 2014, Hasheem Thabeet at 7′3″ and Isaiah Thomas at 5′9″, laid head to foot.

Acquiring the shark alone cost almost $10,000. The entire sculpture cost Saatchi $80,000 in 1990 currency, or $149,000 in today's money, a sum so surprising for a work by an artist then hardly known outside a small circle of young British conceptual artists that the British tabloid *The Sun* ran a story titled "£50,000 for fish without chips."

The shark sculpture is the first of a series of dead and sometimes dissected animals preserved in tanks of formaldehyde that Hirst created over the years. *Mother and Child (Divided)*, for example, consists of a cow and a calf each cut in half and displayed in four glass tanks, the two halves of the calf side by side in front of the similarly placed two halves of the mother. The tanks of each pair have been installed far enough apart for a visitor to walk between them and view the animals' insides. Individually, and even more so collectively, these pieces yank dead animals from behind the walls of factory farms or commercial fisheries in order to force the viewers' acknowledgment that the disembodied, plastic-wrapped animal proteins so ubiquitously consumed by most members of Western societies—including me—actually come from once-living animals.

Hirst's intention in the shark sculpture was to freeze "life and death incarnate" in time by soaking the shark in formaldehyde and injecting it with the preservative liquid until all its natural fluids would be replaced. However, the ancient mummifying technology of exchanging body fluids with a preservative was not successful when applied to an animal as large as Hirst's shark—and some parts were not adequately penetrated. Even as the sculpture's notoriety was building, the shark began to deteriorate, turning the surrounding liquid murky. In an attempt to prolong the work's longevity, the Saatchi gallery added bleach to the formaldehyde solution, which in hindsight was revealed to have sped up the deterioration. In 1993, the decay had become so evident that "the gallery gutted the shark and stretched its skin over a fiberglass mold." Hirst complained that "you could tell it wasn't real."

Despite knowing about the sculpture's lamentable state, in 2004 American hedge fund manager Steven Cohen and his wife

Alexandra bought the piece from Saatchi for $8 million. According to the *New York Times,* "what was floating in the tank was a fiberglass shadow of its former self." Oddly, the shark's tilt from undead to dead appealed to Cohen. "I liked the whole fear factor," he said.

Hirst, however, was not prepared to let go of his original idea. By then he knew that the formaldehyde had not been properly injected and wanted the chance at a do-over. Cohen somewhat reluctantly agreed to trade the "fear factor" for lastingness and even sprung for the replacement of the shark. The process of thoroughly injecting the new carcass alone cost about $100,000. Cohen called the expense "inconsequential." When the operation had been completed, the shark once again cast its Schrödinger's cat smile onto the museum visitors.

However, just as £50,000 failed to permanently incarnate life and death simultaneously in the first "fish without chips," so did $8 million and an inconsequential $100,000 fall short of fixing the second "famous dead shark" in an undead state. In 2006, before commencing a three-year residence in New York City at the Metropolitan Museum of Art, the entire sculpture was refurbished: a new tank and a third new shark were obtained.

Hirst: I would like [*Impossibility*] to always look as fresh as the day I made it, so part of the contract is: if the glass breaks, we mend it; if the tank gets dirty, we clean it; if the shark rots, we find you a new shark. I guarantee my formaldehyde work for 200 years.

Voltaire Cousteau, 200 years ago, "How to Swim with Sharks": DO NOT BLEED. Those who cannot learn to control their bleeding should not attempt to swim with sharks.

Brad Pitt: My theory is, be the shark. You've just got to keep moving.

Hirst: I mean, every day you have to deal with your own mortality, so a good way of doing that without too much fear is to deal with the mortality of an object.

Schrödinger's shark: Being simultaneously dead and alive in the box gave me an incredible perspective over life, the universe, and everything. And I'm here to tell it to the world!

Roberta Smith, *New York Times*: The shark is simultaneously life and death incarnate in a way you don't quite grasp until you see it, suspended and silent, in its tank. It gives the innately demonic urge to live a demonic, deathlike form...It's a reasonable visual metaphor for the crossing-over that we think will never happen.

The crossing-over that we think will never happen. That is, until you have received an approximate expiration date for your own life: terminal cancer, terminal mental decline. From then on, you live every day in the glare of a crossing-over that will happen in a designated time frame. If your diagnosis stems from a physically morbid disease, your focus will likely be on how best to control your pain and other aspects of your journey to death. If your fate is dementia, you focus on the fact by the time the disease has taken you to a "natural" death, your mind will have died long ago. You will have become "simultaneously life and death incarnate." After my dementia diagnosis, I took Hirst's shark very personally: not only *something*, but also *someone* could be there and not there at the same time. And that someone: me.

During my research of Hirst's endless grappling with death in his art—an ongoing project he is still exploring today, long after what he refers to as his "glory days"—I learned that he has for a long time resisted writing an autobiography because it was "an end-of-life activity." By 2015—he is now fifty-one years old—he had started one. Since Hirst is too busy to write his autobiography himself, he has engaged James Fox, who helped Keith Richards of the Rolling Stones with his memoir, as his co-writer.

Hirst himself gives a reason for why he needs a co-writer other than because he is so busy: he can't remember his own past. A large part of Fox's role is to "pluck" anecdotes from interviews with Hirst, together with other sources, to jog the artist's memory. Like Keith Richards, Hirst has "obliterated whole segments of his life." Damien Hirst, too, has entered a state of being there and not there at the same time. "You lose your grip before you die," he said in a recent interview. "I think that's the problem. So I guess [writing a memoir is] how to embrace it in some way."

Dementia Field Notes

8-24-2011

Tonight I accidentally took my own and then Peter's medication. His Simvastatin is twice my dose, so in effect I had taken three doses. Peter and I were supposed to go for fasting blood tests tomorrow, in my case to check my response to the Simvastatin and Lisinopril Dr. Eborn had prescribed to slow down the clogging of the microvessels in my brain. We had to postpone the tests to Friday morning.

On days like this, I always amuse myself by thinking that by the time I overdose on an internet death cocktail—most likely procured with the assistance of my family, but without them actually giving me any help with ingesting it—I will have built up an impressive precedent of medicinal mishaps that should go a long way toward proving that my death was just a plain old miscalculation by a zombie-like addled-pated woman.

"Who am I?"

For those of us acculturated to the Western perception of personhood, the unspoken assumption behind this question is that we

have "a kernel of identity, a self," for example, the self we are encouraged "to get in touch with" or "be true to." When, in graduate
school or otherwise, one is trotted through postmodern concepts
of the self—whether from a philosophical, anthropological, Freudian, or literary critical perspective—you quickly get disabused of
the idea that personhood indicates a single, separate, unified self. A
concept that postmodernist scholars in all of these disciplines have
in common, is that

> the self divides the moment we start looking for it: There
> is the self we're trying to find plus the self that is doing the
> looking plus the self within this game of hide and seek that
> is being played. Even the practice of placing an alarm clock
> out of reach in the bedroom implies that we have at least two
> selves—a responsible nighttime self and a lazy morning self.

In this view, we are not born with a self that merely has to unfold
through the years to reveal our true being, but our self is rather
brought into being by the people we encounter on our life path. Our
self is *relational*, our very self-image is constituted in interactions
with people we have not chosen—not our biological or foster or
adoptive parents, not our first caretakers outside our immediate
family, and not the people in authority we come across in visits to
the pediatrician or witchdoctor, Montessori school or madras, grocery store or street market, church or synagogue.

According to the French psychoanalyst Jacques Lacan, who
interpreted Freud's writings in accordance with anthropological
and linguistic developments that occurred after the father of Psy-
chiatry had died, the symbolic structure of our society—or, "the
Other," to use the phrase in its Lacanian meaning—brings to bear
on us the customs, conventions, and language that define each

individual self. The Other starts shaping a newborn before she has even had the opportunity to develop her own understanding of who she is. The Other, as represented by the family unit at the outset of a child's life, determines the nationality she holds, the languages she speaks, the religious and other values she embraces. While, as an adult, the individual may choose to change her name or conduct her daily life in a language other than her mother tongue or leave behind her family's religion and other values, the influence these factors had on her during her formative years cannot simply be erased. I came out as an atheist to myself when I was seventeen and to everyone else in my twenties, but have nevertheless been shaped by the narratives of the Bible and the white, puritan South African version of Christianity that I had taken in with my mother's milk.

To illustrate the fact that our self is brought into being by the Other, Lacan and other postmodernists refer to a self as a *subject* rather than an *individual,* since the term *individual* arose in the Renaissance to represent the idea that a person could deliberately fashion his own identity. An *individual* is the end result of a person's deliberate and willful manipulation of cultural codes to perfect himself as the person he wants to be. The concept of the individual is equivalent to an idea still bandied about, a way of thinking that I associate with conservative social attitudes: that every *individual* in society should be able to pull herself up by her bootstraps regardless of poverty, social class, or other obstacles toward educational and career achievements. Unlike the concept of the *subject,* this view negates the influence of societal forces on a person's ability to access educational and career opportunities.

Calling someone a "subject" rather than "individual," however, does not imply that the Other only holds back an individual by coercing her to follow communally shared expectations. On the contrary, a term introduced by anthropologist McKim Marriot in 1976, that of the *dividual*, illustrates a form of subjectivity characterized by a deep connection among single persons and their community, bonds achieved through the give and take between single persons and the Other rather than top-down imposition of a mode of being on those persons by the Other.

While the postmodern concept of the dividual dates from the late 1970s, the idea that a self is constituted through other selves is an ancient one. Before the Christian Era, it was embedded in the Buddhist teaching "that anything which depends for its state on external factors must change when those conditioning factors change (*anitya*), and if no part of that thing is immune from dependencies, then to identify any essential protected nucleus of self must be mistaken (*anātman*)." It entered Christianity when the apostle Paul wrote, "we, being many, are one body in Christ, and every one members one of another." It arrived in science with the publication of Carl Linnaeus's *Systema Naturae* in 1753, in which organisms are classified hierarchically into kingdoms, phyla, classes, orders, families, genera, and species based on their structural similarities. Linnaean taxonomy raised "the question: if each species was created separately, as a literal reading of the Bible would imply, why were there structural similarities across species, genera, classes, etc.? Why was Linnaeus' classification sensible?"

A century later, Charles Darwin answered the question Linnaeus's work had raised with the publication of *On the Origin of Species*. Darwin proposed natural selection as the mechanism that made possible the evolution of trilobytes to tree ferns and hadrosaurs to hominids from primitive life forms that appeared on earth 3.5 billion years ago. Once the concept of the dividual entered the realm of living organisms, it took just "one small step for a man, one giant leap for mankind" before it was extended to non-living material objects all through the universe. Dividuality rings from Carl Sagan's praise song to the Universe in the TV series *Cosmos*: "The beauty of a living thing is not only the atoms that go into it, but the way those atoms are put together. The cosmos is also within us. We're made of star stuff. We are a way for the cosmos to know itself." It reverberates in Neil deGrasse Tyson's desire "to grab people in the street and say, 'Have you heard this? The molecules in my body are traceable to phenomena in the cosmos.'"

In its route from Buddhism through Christianity, the biological sciences, postmodernist thinking, and astronomy, the "self" has become multiplicitous and heterogeneous and never complete—it is, rather, ceaselessly becoming.

The answer to "Who am I?" has gained—or regained—cosmic proportions.

There are those—ranging from conservative Christians to humanities scholars of all stripes—who don't like this "self" that cannot be pinned down. The former believe that the postmodern self is "a revolution against the God of the Bible" by "people no longer willing to comply with God's guidelines [who] want to be free to do as they please" and the latter that it leaves single persons "bereft of origin and purpose."

The postmodernist self resonates with the way I experience myself. I'm never done; always changing; dependent on external factors that include people, events, and the matter of which my body consists; and, more often than not, not under the sway of reason. In this framework, "Who am I?" can never be fully answered. "Know thyself" is a shadow on the wall of Plato's cave. However, in a universe that can mathematically be described as the three-dimensional shadow caused by the collapse of a four-dimensional star that resulted in the Big Bang, a shadow gives us a lot to work with: in the same way that astronomers read the history of the universe down to when it was only a hundredth of a billionth of a trillionth of a trillionth of a second old, the postmodern subject can be read "through its discourse, its actions, its being with other selves, and its experience of transcendence."

In the meantime, I cling to my dividuality for *self*-ish reasons that would better befit a Renaissance *in*dividual. In *The Village Effect: How Face-to-Face Contact Can Make Us Healthier, Happier, and Smarter*, developmental psychologist and journalist Susan Pinker cites neuroscience findings showing that "those who avoid dementia have the most complex and integrated social network."

Dementia Field Notes

11-10-2011

Peter and I are visiting Marissa and Adam in Chicago. Last night Marissa, Peter, and I were in the living room examining life in our usual jokingly serious way. Our topic, what would happen to Peter if I died before him. Adam was doing homework at his desk in the corner.

Gerda: You'd better get a second wife.

Peter: The kids will be far too fussy to accept anyone as my second wife.

Gerda: The kids will be all too happy if you have your own company because else they have to deal with you being lonely and miserable.

Marissa: The problem is, Dad, that your second wife will have to be able to talk technology and be interested in your electronic toys—

Gerda: Unlike me.

Marissa: I have an idea. We should outsource Dad's second wife to India.

We all elaborated on the idea of Peter finding a tech-savvy immigrant from India or anywhere else where someone might be interested in a "green card" marriage.

Gerda: Those women can still cook. Maybe you can come to an arrangement of a number of years in which she would cook and care for you as "payment" for the green card and then go on with her own life.

Peter: I love Indian food. But what about sex?

"Sex" pops Adam out of his homework. He swivels his chair all the better to not miss a word.

Gerda: That can be in the contract or not. What do I care?

Peter: Maybe I love Mexican food even more.

Gerda: As long as you don't exploit one of my fabulous undocumented former students.

Peter: But Layla* told us that her father always says, "Why do you fall in love with an undocumented boy? You should fall in love with someone who can make you legal!"

Marissa: Mom, I think your last testament should require that Dad's second wife must be older than me.

––––––––

On the day his father finally died of Alzheimer's disease, novelist Jonathan Franzen noted that "in the slow-motion way of Alzheimer's, my father wasn't much deader now than he had been two hours or two weeks or two months ago." Franzen is by no means the only relative of a dementia sufferer who has thought of his loved one as, in effect, dead while he was still alive. "Undead," to be succinct. Not surprisingly, then, both scholarly and popular writing frequently refer to persons with dementia as zombies.

––––––––

* Not her real name.

In an essay titled "The Living Dead? The Construction of People with Alzheimer's Disease as Zombies," political scientist Susan Behuniak draws attention to the use of "the 'undead' metaphor" for people with dementia, which, she argues, magnifies the stigmatization already visited on such patients by the biomedical model of the disease. This model, she claims, positions someone with dementia "as a non-person, i.e. one whose brain has been destroyed by the disease and who therefore no longer exists as a person but only as a body to be managed."

In a survey of scholarly and popular writings about dementia, Behuniak notes that dementia is referred to, for example, as "death before death," "the funeral that never ends," "the mind robber," and "a terror-inspiring plague." Such observations are frequently directly connected with the term *zombie* as well. She goes on to compile a list of characteristics shared by zombies and people who have dementia, which includes "exceptional physical characteristics, lack of self-recognition, failure to recognize others, cannibalization of human beings... [and] overwhelming hopelessness that makes death a preferred alternative than [*sic*] continued existence." She concedes that these attributes are accurate in describing people with dementia, since they often have a disheveled and badly groomed physical appearance and shuffling walk and are given to obsessive wandering. In regard to zombie cannibalism, she cites examples of a dementia patient who refers to his disease as "'the closest thing to being eaten alive slowly'" and another who says in relation to his caretakers that "'the unique curse of Alzheimer's Disease (AD) is that it ravages several victims for every brain it infects.'"

Behuniak's examples come from publications that, like she does, advocate more humane treatment of dementia patients, such as nursing and gerontology journals and writings by AD sufferers themselves or their relatives. She emphasizes that the purpose of her essay is to show that language is a powerful social force that has been and is still used to set apart those among us who lack some essential aspects of what society believes "a full human being" should look like. The result is that those who do not qualify are deemed not worthy of the full self-determination to which "normal" people feel themselves entitled.

Given my lifelong love affair with language and having taught the major civil rights battles of the past century in my Gender Studies courses, I am aware of the role language has played in the efforts of disenfranchised communities to gain full civil rights. Activists in the various movements have invariably regarded a campaign against language used derogatorily against their group as a necessary part of their fight. The almost total elimination from polite language of the n-word, "bitch," "queer," "cripple," and so on attests to their success. Given the unruly nature of language, however, some have reclaimed the former derogatory words as badges of honor but always with the clear expectation that only some people have a "right" to these words. Since I myself am walking the teetering plank toward the neither-dead-nor-alive identity of someone with dementia, I have some things to say about Behuniak's proposed banishment of "zombie" in this context. First, though, a confession: I know hardly anything about zombies through firsthand experience. I have never seen a whole zombie movie. The visual image the word evokes in my head derives from a handful of YouTube clips.

How the topic of zombies came up during a discussion in one of my Gender Studies classes, I do not remember. However, what is clearly imprinted in my memory is that a young man at the back of the room, who hardly ever spoke, corrected me when I had apparently used vampires and zombies interchangeably. That I had made an impression on my student, albeit a negative one, became evident at the next meeting of the class. To encouraging hoots and clapping from the other students, he presented me with my own copy of *The Zombie Survival Guide*, which I of course accepted with all the grace I could muster.

It had been a matter of pride for me to read—or at least skim—the whole book before the next class so that I could at least redeem myself with an informed comment or two. To my surprise, I found Max Brooks's fiction more interesting than its literary forebears. It also fascinated me that George Romero's genre-inventing film, *Night of the Living Dead*, had gone completely by me when it debuted in 1968 when I was in the middle of my BS degree at the University of Pretoria and that *Dead Alive*, which came out in 1992 when I was in the middle of my English PhD, had passed me like a ship in the night. I had clearly not been on the zombie ward's phone list.

The book was a glimpse into a cult the existence of which I had never heard of—lovers of the zombie genre who particularly delight in the humor and self-mocking of a kinder, gentler new zombiehood, in which even Disney's Ariel and Snow White are zombie princesses. Such, then, is the background against which I declare myself a zombie princess in waiting. I put my dibs on the name "Princess Doña Quixote."

Setting aside my compensatory attempts at humor, I want to talk about something that bothered me in Behuniak's essay, namely her characterization of the biomedical model of dementia as necessarily evil. First, her definition does not at all accord with those one finds in medical dictionaries and scholarly medical and psychiatric articles. For example, MedicineNet defines dementia as a disease that leads to "significant loss of intellectual abilities, such as memory capacity, that is severe enough to interfere with social or occupational functioning," and the National Collaborating Centre for Mental Health as "a clinical syndrome characterised by global cognitive impairment, which represents a decline from previous level of functioning, and is associated with impairment in functional abilities and, in many cases, behavioural and psychiatric disturbances."

It seems to me that Behuniak's misrepresentation and disapproval of the biomedical model is the result of a categorical confusion. Philosophy, and its application in the sciences when it comes to the meaning of words, distinguishes between two different kinds of definitions: descriptive, which depict a state of affairs, and normative, which delineates the ethical action that derives from a state of affairs. The definitions of the biomedical model that I reproduced above are descriptive and not normative. Normative expectations derived from a state of dementia, or how we should act toward people with dementia, abound in the very nursing and other medical literature from which Behuniak derives her examples of what a climate of care *should* look like in relation to dementia. Such normative definitions are known as biopsychosocial models and are similar to those advanced by Thomas Kitwood and the other personal-centered theorists Behuniak cites: they advocate approaches to dementia that assume "the person is present and approaches AD as a condition shaped and defined by the social and interpersonal contexts rather than by neurological changes alone."

Despite the widespread adoption during the 1980s of the biopsychosocial model of "health"—including "health" in the context of brain-destroying diseases—by large medical organizations in the United States as well as other countries where Western medicine is practiced, the change of language has not yet permeated a large enough part of medical practice, though it has made many inroads. The problem in the case of dementia caretaking, therefore, can be ascribed to a lack of financial resources for training and paying living wages as much as to negative language.

As someone who puts a *physical, material* understanding of my disease at the top of my conceptual hierarchy, I take the descriptive definition of brain disease very seriously. It is precisely the focus on physical, material investigations of the human brain that has enabled the remarkable knowledge base currently being assembled faster than even experts in the neurological field can absorb it. As evidence I present the July/August edition of the *MIT Technology Review*—one of the science magazines I read during visits to the bathroom—the entire issue of which is dedicated to "new technologies that look inside the mind [and] will make it possible to change what we think, feel, and remember." The issue is titled "Hacking the Soul."

Rather than the biggest fear Behuniak ascribes to people with dementia—to be "dehumanized through social construction as the 'living dead'"—my biggest fear is that dementia will be eating a large enough portion of my already non-normal-appearing and -functioning neurons, glial cells, blood vessels, and other brain constituents that it won't be possible for me to opt out of a zombie existence by myself and on my own terms, a fear that will probably cause me to err on the side of prematurity as I plan for my eventual suicide.

Dementia Field Notes

11-28-2011

We went to the gym and I walked 3-something miles on the track with Susan. I forgot that my green exercise shoes hurt me and accidentally put them on. I got bad bunion blisters from when I ran a few laps.

While walking and talking with Susan, I was making a point about shrinking and growing friendships and several times forgot what point I was trying to make during a monologue. Fortunately, when I write I can go back and retrace my logic and eventually get together an argument. I find myself increasingly at a loss to participate in spoken conversations.

———————

One of the first things Peter and I investigated after my dementia diagnosis was long-term care. We knew that it was very expensive, and we were willing to give up some of our retirement dreams, such as regular trips to South Africa while I could still travel, to make it possible. However, it did not take long to discover that once a person has had any kind of memory tests, you can no longer qualify for long-term-care insurance. Not even under Obamacare. Long-term-care insurance falls under the laws that regulate, for example, fire, earthquake, or car insurance rather than medical insurance. In other words, you can legally be refused for "pre-existing conditions" such as living in a house made exclusively out of wood or one in a seismic zone, having a bad driving record, or having had memory difficulties. Up to a point, extraordinary amounts of money can buy this kind of insurance, except in the case of long-term care. Once you've had any memory-related issues, even queries to your doctor that did not result in a follow-up but made it into your doctor's notes, you cannot buy long-term care at any price. Fortunately Peter qualified for such care and we immediately bought a policy. Since it was a certainty that I was not going to be able to take care of him should he become debilitated, his having long-term insurance has given me much peace of mind.

During July 2014, we discovered that my memory tests have disqualified me from another insurance possibility we had been pursuing, a policy known as "hospital indemnity" that pays out to help

cover medical costs requiring hospitalization or a time in a rehabilitation facility.

Given these realities, Peter and I now know that we will have to
deal with my mental regression through Medicare, supplemented
by whatever of our own retirement savings we will be able to shave
off as well as the moral support of our children, their families, and
the rest of our village.

Dementia Field Notes

12-10-2011

We are on the plane to New York for Peter's office Christmas
party. Since he is a consultant working from home, it did not at
all occur to him that Constratus would have a Christmas party.
However, his boss called a few days ago to say that he was going
to fly both Peter and me to NYC and put us up in the downtown
Marriott for the whole weekend so that we could attend the party
on Sunday. The party is three hours out of the city, so Mr. Nice
arranged a limousine ride for us too.

As we were settling in on the plane earlier, I closed one of
the seatbelt-like clips on my gray travel bag without incident.
When I got to the second one, though, instead of picking up the
lower part of the clip I gripped the zipper tag and tried to stick
it into the top half of the clip. Peter was watching and from his
concerned expression I could see that he, too, had a moment of
realization that some of my dementia issues are progressing faster
than we (I) thought they would.

When we were in Chicago in October, I asked Marissa if
I could borrow her book *Final Exit: The Practicalities of Self-
Deliverance and Assisted Suicide for the Dying*. I have been

reading it for future reference, but I just realized that I had better seriously figure out the end plan sooner rather than later, while a considerable part of my brain still works. Not that I plan a speedy exit, but just to have all the necessary discussions with Peter and the children and draw up a guide for Peter and the kids when the right time comes. In the end it will be their decision whether to assist me in my suicide (only in ways that are legal) or warehouse my emptied-out-head-attached-to-my-life-clinging-body until my strong heart stops.

In August 2014, our family celebrated thirty years of living in our adopted country. The American Saunderses have grown to nine people: Newton's wife, Cheryl, has now been part of our family for going on fifteen years, and Marissa's husband, Adam, for five. Newton and Cheryl's two children, Kanye and Aliya, are seven and four, respectively—the same ages Marissa and Newton were when we emigrated. Marissa and Adam have eighteen-month-old Dante. Once Cheryl and Adam had gotten over the shock of our family's no-topic-barred habits around each other, they have been giving us a taste of our own medicine.

None of the adults in our family regards themselves as religious, and the grandkids will decide for themselves as they grow older. Among the six adults, our ethical frameworks and other life principles are similar in broad strokes. Both our children and their spouses are as open to their children's hows and whys as Peter and I were when our children were young, except that they seem to have less angst than we had. (We were, after all, blazing a trail out of our own upbringings of "children are seen and not heard.") As an extended family, then, we had done much of the prep that should ideally precede the open discussion of my dementia.

Though the questions we launched into after my prognosis were personal and focused on me, the conceptual ground involved was already familiar to us, since we had had similar conversations when Cheryl's grandfather was fitted with a feeding tube in his nineties and lived miserably for three more years. So, again, we asked: What is a quality of life or degree of incapacitation each of us would find acceptable? How would we like to spend the last year or month of our lives? What if one of us is no longer capable of rational decision making and is miserable all the time while her body is still in relatively good working order? What quality of long-term care is available for a dementia sufferer of my and Peter's financial means through Medicare and private funds? How do we feel about last-ditch life-extending efforts, and what would their financial and psychic consequences be for each of our three family units? Under what conditions would each of us commit suicide or seek an assisted death? How would each of us feel or react if one of the others wanted to end their lives before their bodies gave in?

While Peter and I have for many years declared a theoretical position that favors the compassionate ending of a life versus years of misery, we now tackled the concept as a practical reality. Our children hold the same theoretical positions and now declared their practical support to put a suicide plan in place for me. And so started our investigation into the practicalities and legalities of suicide and assisted suicide. Peter and I were of course adamant about not asking our children to participate in actions that would expose them to investigation or prosecution.

In the months—now years—that followed, I surveyed the right-to-die landscape while the rest of my family kept their ears and eyes open and sent me links, articles, or anecdotes as they happened upon them. My research revealed that (1) whatever scant legal or at least non-prosecutable opportunities exist for citizens in our own country to die with dignity do not extend to someone with a terminal mental disease, since the five right-to-die states—Oregon, Washington, Vermont, Montana, and New Mexico—all require two doctors' declarations that the person seeking death would likely die within six months *and is of sound mind*. Since dementia patients are by definition no longer of sound mind by the time their disease will have driven them insane, American end-of-life laws in their present form will not be of any benefit to our family; (2) the legal landscape is rapidly changing. Even where the laws remain unaltered, popular sympathy for families who resort to assisted death has made prosecution very unlikely—no one has been convicted or had to serve a prison term for assisting in a suicide since 1998, not even Dr. Kevorkian. He was acquitted of assisted suicide three times in jury trials.

The absence of overtly "technological" or "medical" means in most assisted deaths seems to be the key to why so few family members who have assisted a relative in dying by pulverizing lethal drugs and making a cocktail out of them have been successfully prosecuted, or even prosecuted at all. The last case prosecuted that I could find was that of Barbara Mancini, a Philadelphia nurse who did no more than hand her still-rational, terminally ill, ninety-three-year-old father a nearly full bottle of morphine. He drank it while she was no longer in the room. He was "saved from himself" by a hospice nurse who called 911. Four days later he died at the hospital.

Even though Mancini was eventually acquitted, a year-long investigation and trial had forced her to take "unpaid leave from her nursing job" and she incurred "more than $100,000 in legal fees." Her husband, Joe Mancini, "had taken on extra paramedic shifts to help supplement the family's income." Of course, the last thing a person asking relatives to assist her in dying wants is to expose the people they love most in the world to such horrible consequences.

In October 2014, Brittany Maynard, a twenty-nine-year-old woman who had been diagnosed with terminal brain cancer and decided to end her life through physician-assisted death (PAD), significantly advanced public understanding and acceptance of dying people to choose the time and manner of their own death. "Mature and savvy beyond her years," Maynard contacted Compassion and Choices, a national advocacy group for legalizing end-of-life choices, to offer her story in their support. She had by then teamed up with a filmmaker and gone on camera to describe her disease and explain her family's choice to move to Oregon, where PAD was legal, because her home state of California did not offer her the possibility of a self-determined death.

Once Compassion and Choices had released Maynard's video statement, her story generated international attention. Young, attractive, eloquent, and supported by a loving family, she succeeded in making many people see PAD not as an outré possibility for a special class of hard-hearted families, but as something they might choose themselves. Her grace and dignity, together with the bravery of her mother and husband, who endorsed her decision even as their hearts were breaking, drew an unprecedented flood of empathy and support that persisted after her death on November 1, 2014, and resulted in the passing of a right-to-die law in California less than a year later. According to the leading journal of health policy thought and research, *Health Affairs*, her case might result in additional states considering right-to-die legislation: "Predictions that, by the end of the year, 26 states will be seriously considering PAD legislation do not seem outlandish."

In the context of dementia, do-it-yourself death options through organizations such as Compassion and Choices and the Death with

Dignity National Center are not very encouraging. Given that, even in states where PAD is legal, one has to execute all acts relating to your death by yourself, most dementia sufferers will likely not be able to follow through without help from a family member once they are in the advanced stages of the disease. If I already have difficulty setting out my weekly medications in a compartmentalized dispenser and taking the correct day's pills, how will I manage ten, fifteen years from now to obtain, pulverize, and mix the lethal drugs for my final sundowner without substantial help from my family? Since I now already have to ask Peter to always check if I have combed my hair before we go out the door, how will I be able to set up a tank of helium and place the tube inside the plastic bag I am supposed to fix in a leak-proof manner around my head? Although I really do not want to have an undead existence, I value my family members' legal indemnity more than my wish for self-determination, even though they themselves at this time feel that, from an ethical and practical perspective, they would want to help me die. For me to realize my preference for a physician-assisted suicide, then, I investigated yet another option: traveling to Europe to obtain a legal death there.

There are indeed ways for foreigners to seek a dignified death in certain European countries. While the last thing a person with advanced dementia needs is an overseas trip, I would want to go through with it if that were the way to spare myself from zombiehood and my family years of taking care of a pale shade of who I used to be. Should the possibility arise to obtain an assisted death closer to home, we would all very much prefer that. However, US states where assisted death is legal have made it almost impossible for "outsiders" to get an assisted death, though internet rumors suggest there might be ways around it. We have set no hopes on Utah making assisted death legal in any of our lifetimes, including those of our grandchildren. Unless there is a change in the zeitgeist that brings assisted death closer to our "pretty, great state," Peter and our children have declared themselves game to undertake "the death trip" to Europe with me.

Dividuality? My family defines it.

Dementia Field Notes

3-3-2012

This morning I accidentally took my evening medication—the morning and evening pills are in two different, clearly marked dispensers.

I'm now sitting in the Columbus Community Center's library. I brought [the daughter of one of our neighbors] to sign up for an art activity to be held in the summer. The person teaching it is a professor at the U whose art we had used on a Women's Week poster many years ago—she depicts fabulous women of color in superwoman outfits and poses. Since the project is for kids older than the girl, I came to ask the artist to make an exception. She is in.

After finishing this entry, I am going to read *Final Exit*. I wrapped it in Billy Collins's *Nine Horses* cover, because in this setting I do not want to advertise my suicide. If it were not for the kids around, I would of course have flaunted it in public, since death with dignity is an issue whose time has come.

Peter and I put our end-of-life-plans, including the death trip, on paper with a lawyer's help. After we did, I learned about a method of suicide that seems more feasible to our family than what we had already described in our legal documents. The beauty is that its implementation does not require any legal dancing around. The method is voluntarily stopping eating and drinking, dubbed VSED by the medical community.

Cheryl was the one who sent me an article about it, a piece by Nell Lake, a reporter who focuses on the care of people at the end of their lives. The piece, "Aid-in-Dying Loophole: Advocates Want You to Know You Can Stop Eating and Drinking," posted on the website for WBUR, the Boston NPR station, tells the story of a daughter helping her mother with advanced dementia to stop eating and drinking. It comforts me to know that someone in whose shoes I am walking, albeit some distance behind, was able to muster the discipline to stick to a plan that requires the mental stamina to overcome the instant gratification of food and drink.

Jackie Wilton had lived with dementia for several years before she sought a diagnosis and another "few years" afterward. In the spring of 2012, when Jackie was eighty-four years old, she first explicitly asked her daughter Kathleen Klein to help her die. Fiercely independent all her life, Jackie was deeply disturbed by having to rely on Kathleen for just about every daily activity. Her request did not come out of the blue. After her diagnosis Jackie had frequently spoken of dying on her own terms before she became severely incapacitated. Though Kathleen and her sister and brother had known about their mother's intention, they had never discussed a particular mode of suicide. Accordingly, when Jackie first asked Kathleen for help, the latter had no idea how to go about assisting her mother to die or even whether she was willing to risk the threat of prosecution. Not long after that first conversation, though, Kathleen heard a radio interview about "voluntary stopping of eating or drinking," or VSED. It was "the only legal form of assisted suicide" and was increasingly being advocated by death-with-dignity advocates. Besides being legal, VSED is a naturally occuring symptom of the death process in people dying over a long period, and accordingly something with which medical professionals and other caretakers of the dying are familiar.

Given that suicide is not a crime in the United States and that VSED is frequently used by mentally competent terminally ill patients to hasten their death, it sounded like a viable option. Kathleen discovered that Medicare would provide hospice support as soon as Jackie had stopped eating and drinking long enough to be in pain, unable to get out of bed, or have lost 10 percent of her body weight. After she met any one of these criteria, a doctor would be able to declare that she would likely die within six months. Hospice would then immediately kick in.

Jackie agreed to stop eating and drinking. Kathleen describes her mother's dying on a blog post written after her death.

After letting her siblings know about Jackie's decision, Kathleen and her mother got started. Jackie asked what the rules were so that she could keep them. They agreed that should Jackie ask for something to eat or drink, Kathleen would remind her of her goal. If Jackie wanted to continue VSED, Kathleen would keep withholding food and drink. If she decided she no longer wanted to continue, Kathleen would give her whatever she wanted.

Mother and daughter rolled out the plan with a drastic reduction in Jackie's oral intake—a few spoons of yogurt and up to a cup of water per day. Although she rapidly lost weight and strength, after almost two weeks she was still far from death. She was disappointed every morning when she realized she was still alive. As the days passed, Jackie and Kathleen spent time looking at old photographs so that Jackie could pick one for her obituary. The dying woman picked one where she was about sixteen or seventeen. "I suppose she felt more like that was her real life," Kathleen writes, "not the one she had now."

Once the drastic cut in Jackie's intake had been established, Kathleen's sister arrived and, soon after, her brother and his children. Jackie's doctor came to visit, too. Although he was against all forms of suicide, he set aside his own convictions and supported his long-time patient. Paying a house call four days into the plan, he told Kathleen that Jackie would have to stop all eating and drinking to ensure that her dying would not stretch out longer than two to three weeks. From then on, Kathleen gave Jackie only "quarter-sized ice chips" in very limited quantity.

On the seventh day, Kathleen's brother said goodbye. After he had left, Jackie no longer left her bedroom. She complained of pain and Kathleen called the hospice. They went out to Jackie's home and gave her morphine. By this time the dying woman's mouth was already constantly dry, and a side effect of morphine was that it increased thirst. Recalling "an old Indian trick" her brother had told her about in childhood, Kathleen picked a small shiny rock out of the glass bowl in which Jackie had displayed the smooth stones and offered it to her mother. It worked and she sucked it for the rest of the time that she was awake. On the ninth day, Jackie went into a coma. On the thirteenth day, she died.

Kathleen ends her blog post with a reflection on the day of Jackie's death. "The sun was shining in Morrow Bay. There was a light breeze. It was a day that, at one time, she would have enjoyed being out in, going for a drive or taking a walk."

Reflection on Journal Entry of 5-24-2012

I have been too busy to write for a long time now—I see it is over two months since I last got to it. I feel anxious and frustrated because of not writing and am really aware of good brain time ticking by, since the multiple ways my brain is failing are more evident when I am stressed and tired.

We are now at Hurricane, near Zion National Park, with Newton, Cheryl, and their kids. Peter says—and I agree—that this is a vacation in which he feels very much loved. Newton and Cheryl are so considerate and loving, and Kanye and Aliya stimulating company. It is very gratifying to see that as my brain disintegrates, theirs are growing exponentially.

We were all so happy to get the news on our way here that Marissa is pregnant. The baby is due in late January of next year. Of course, giving the kind of time to a grandchild that I do will also reduce my writing time—but attentive time with my grandkids is the one thing I never regret spending time on.

One of the stress mistakes I made happened on Friday night when we arrived here. I was getting something in the car and was disoriented in space. I put my hand where I thought the seat was, but missed—so I fell out of the car. I felt shocked and embarrassed, particularly because I screamed while going down. I think I was more upset than I usually am about such a small thing because of a childhood incident when I was about seven or eight and we were living in the house by Oom Koot and Tannie Wienkie.

Some of my siblings and I were outside waiting for Ma to stop talking to Tannie Wienkie because we were going to drive somewhere. In boredom, Klasie and I started climbing in and out of the windows. At some point I was hanging out of the open window backwards, managing to stay up by gripping the window's sides. My hands must have been sweaty, because they slowly slipped downward. I knew my grip was going to fail soon and I started screaming. Ma was probably so used to kids screaming that she did not react. I fell to the ground. I got a scrape on my arm and a bump on my head. While I felt sorry for myself at the time, in hindsight I feel sorrier for my mother—she was visibly upset that she had not paid attention to me. The irony is that even as a child I knew that my mother paid us much more of what I now think of as creative attention than any of the other farm mothers I knew: she hung a display board covered with a burlap bag near our front door where we nailed curly acacia pods, a twig of particularly large thorns, flowers we found in the veld, and mouse skeletons.

———————

After rehearsing our end-of-life ideas with our children for about two years, Peter and I were ready to formalize them legally. In spring 2013, we discussed our situation with our doctor and a lawyer we had selected for his openness about pursuing the legal and financial implications of assisted suicide. During the months-long process of our lawyer's and our own ongoing research into legal possibilities, we updated our children with every piece of new information. For example, we learned that it is possible for people who have a physical illness that is terminal and are of sound mind to move to a state where assisted death is legal (i.e., Oregon, Vermont, Washington, New Mexico, and Montana), fulfill their minimum duration of residency requirement, and apply for physician assisted death—an option that still excluded people like me. However, our lawyer obtained the contact information of a doctor in a different state (possibly connected to a network of like-minded physicians) who would be willing to prescribe a suicide cocktail so that one would not have to deal with the internet.

Once our lawyer had drafted the necessary documents, we met with him as a family—Peter, Newton, and I attended the meeting at the lawyer's office in person; Cheryl joined in by video from South Jordan where they live; and so did Marissa and Adam from Chicago. While projecting the relevant pages of our documents, he laid out the trust fund he had set up together with our financial advisor for expenses related to my assisted death. It provides for the Saunders adults' "death trip" to Europe.

No one cried in the lawyer's office that day. The crying, for this phase of our plans, was behind us. There were times when we laughed: hearing the substance of our dining table discussions over the past years put into legalese was funny. It was like signing the papers for a house after you've done all the legwork and are ready to commit to a three-decade mortgage. The anticipation of the family bonds that would grow still stronger in the space your family is about to inhabit more than compensates for the leaky pipes, the broken furnace, and the stuck windows that are as inevitable as death.

When our lawyer started the meeting, there were no surprises, just a fleshing out of already familiar concepts. When we got to our advanced health care directives, he explained that Peter and I had given both our children as well as each of their spouses power of attorney to act as our agents in end-of-life decisions. With the relevant pages of our last will and testament and advanced health care directives projected on a wall screen and a computer whiteboard, he talked us all through the fine print. During our discussion of the health care directives, he showed a statement I had drafted and he had translated into legal language in order to expand the powers of our "health care agents" (i.e., our children) as they relate to my and Peter's separate, individual wishes to have an assisted death. It is titled "An Acceptable Quality of Life in the Context of Dementia" and here are parts of it.

> In addition to avoiding [mental and physical] suffering, a worthwhile life should include the qualities of joy, acceptance, "being with family, having the touch of others, being mentally aware, and not becoming a burden to others." A life without

these qualities results in an unacceptable quality of life. Death is as much a reality as birth, growth, maturity and old age; however, it should not include the indignity of useless deterioration, dependence and hopeless pain. Therefore, I have executed this Directive in part to relieve all feelings of guilt or responsibility for my death for my Agent and loved ones. I intend that my family, any person to whom I have granted the power to provide informed consent for health care decisions on my behalf, my physicians and their medical assistants, my lawyer and any medical facility caring for me and its personnel cooperate with me and with each other in carrying out my directions and in allowing me to die with dignity, by the use of euthanasia and/or assisted suicide for my person, if and when I do not have an acceptable quality of life.

I direct that upon my request or upon the request of any Agent designated by me with the power to make health care decisions, that physicians assist me in my dying so that I may die in a dignified, painless, and humane manner.

I would like my friends and relatives to regard the following circumstances as flags that the quality of life I want to have is dwindling below the level of acceptability, whether I am at that point still at home or in a care center:

- Do I wake up most days feeling joyful and excited about my new day, no matter the level of intellectual activity I am capable of?
- Do I look forward to more things than I dread?
- Do I appear and act happy for more hours per day than I appear and act unhappy?
- Do I complain frequently about loneliness, depression, or boredom?

- Do I sleep most of the day?
- Am I insatiable in my needs and demands of my caretakers, be they family or care center personnel?
- Does it take my combined caretakers more hours per day to care for me than the hours when I am not consuming care?
- Should I be at home, is/are my primary caretaker(s) stressed and worn out and constantly on the edge of a breakdown?
- Do I enjoy being in my garden (or that of the care center) watching the plants, birds, insects? Can I physically get there without needing a team of people?
- Are my caretakers' children or jobs or quality of life suffering as a result of their care for me?
- Do my family members feel I am still within the boundaries of a meaningful life as they have seen me living it over the years?
- Do I give comfort to my friends, children, and grandchildren, or am I disturbed by their presence and suspicious of their intentions?
- Do I revert to the racism I learned as a child in apartheid South Africa (as my mother did)?
- Am I physically approachable without getting myself into a state of fear or anger; that is, is it still a pleasure for me to cuddle with a friend or child or grandchild? In other words, do I still provide (and enjoy) "the comfort of a warm body"?

In our lawyer's office, after everybody's remaining questions—there were hardly any—had been asked and answered, Peter and I signed the documents. On the way home, our conversation was an iteration, through various memories and anecdotes, that we were the luckiest parents in the world.

*   *   *

Physicist Enrico Fermi left a legacy far more positive than his eventual reluctant participation toward building Little Boy and Fat Man, the two fission bombs that ended the Second World War: the so-called "Fermi Questions," physics puzzles he devised to teach students how to rapidly estimate a quantity that is either difficult or impossible to measure directly. One of Fermi's questions has attained cult status among physics and chemistry aficionados—a cult to which I belong. The puzzle is known as "the last breath of Caesar": When you take a single breath, how many molecules of your gas intake would come from the dying breath of Julius Caesar?

Fermi taught his students how to find a back-of-the-envelope answer in a few minutes by combining their general knowledge of the world and basic principles of physics. In the case of Caesar's last breath, you already know the approximate radius of Earth; the formula for the volume of a sphere; the number of atoms in a liter of gas, namely Loschmidt's number, or 2.687×10^{19}; the molecular masses of the major components of the atmosphere, oxygen and nitrogen; and so on. Using this information, it is easy to calculate the answer: every time I breathe in, there is a good chance that at least one of the molecules I take into my lungs will have been sighed out on the Ides of March, 44 BCE, by Gaius Julius Caesar, at that very moment, causing "the herds of horses which he had dedicated to the river Rubicon when he crossed it, [to] stubbornly refuse to graze and weep copiously."

As I prepare for the day—even though I think it may still be years in the future—when I will tell my family and friends, like Caesar did after his triumphal march in Rome, that "I have lived long enough to satisfy both nature and glory," the whimsy of Caesar's last breath thrills me with the promise it contains of a connection between the material world, where my constituent parts will dwell after my death, and the world of the living, now and ever more—or, at least, the ever-more until our universe comes to an end.

The story I tell myself about my place in the universe—before I was born, now, and after I die—centers on my part in a grand cycle, of which my conscious life is but "a small parenthesis in eternity." Like all grand narratives about the meaning of one's life, mine is a bricolage of found tales, some of which I have kept as is because of their vintage, poetic charm, and others that I have refurbished for my own particular tastes. Here are a few cornerstones of my poly-angular personal manifesto about "The Meaning of Life":

Genesis: In the beginning...the earth was without form, and void; and darkness was upon the face of the deep. And the Spirit of God moved upon the face of the waters.

Exodus: In the beginning, the universe was very small and very hot. Within minutes of the Big Bang explosion, atomic particles came together to make the simple elements.*

Numbers: "Many African societies divide humans into three cat-egories: [those] still alive on the earth,...The recently departed whose time on·earth overlapped with people still here..., the living-dead. They are not wholly dead, for they still live in the memories of the living, who can call them to mind, create their likenesses in art, and bring them to life in an anecdote. When the last person to know an ancestor dies, that ancestor leaves the...[living dead] for [category 3] the dead....As generalized ancestors,...[the dead] are not forgotten but revered...But they are not the living-dead. There is a difference."

Psalms:

In the beginning was the word, the word
that from the solid bases of the light

---

* Big Bang story I told my children and now tell my grandchildren.

abstracted all the letters of the void;
and from the cloudy bases of the breath
the word flowed up, translating to the heart
first characters of birth and death.

Song of Solomon: "The very molecules that make up your body, the atoms that construct the molecules, are traceable to the crucibles that were once the centers of high-mass stars that exploded their chemically rich guts into the galaxy, enriching pristine gas clouds with the chemistry of life. So that we are all connected: to each other biologically, to the earth chemically, and to the rest of the universe atomically."

Acts: Existence precedes essence. There is no essence, or meaning to life, before human existence: living is a biological drive, that's what cells do. We have to create such essence in time and in concrete, irremediably unique circumstances. We ourselves have to endow our lives with meaning. As Sartre puts it in *Existentialism Is a Humanism*, "man first of all exists, encounters himself, surges up in the world—and defines himself afterwards...Man is, before all else, something which propels itself towards a future and is aware of doing so. Man is, indeed, a project."

Revelation: Thus spake Doña Quixote: My village, without which I would have no self-definition, reaches from our red front door to the event horizon of our universe, that shielding cloak outside of which the laws of physics no longer hold. My consciousness, that small parenthesis, is confined between the moment my developing brain had its first input from my senses-in-progress and the moment I can no longer conceive of my village or its inhabitants. In each moment of this wild and precious life, "the future coils, / a tree inside a pit. Take, / eat, we are each other's / perfection."

By the time I, like the rest of my fifteen million mind-addled Baby Boomer buddies, cross from being alive to the living death of madness—that is, when people will rightly say "Gerda is no longer Gerda"—the pre-mad Gerda will be relocated from the diseased matter of her brain to the hale and hearty minds of her earthly kin, those to whom she had grappled herself with hooks of steely love, there evermore to dwell in their keep, evermore ensconced in "the holiness of [their] hearts' affections"—or at least for the evermore that will last until they, too, become either one of the zombie-style "living dead."

Madam, there is only one exit: madness and death.

A categorical overlap bridges the living dead and the wholly dead. This intersection is a material one; it happens on the level of molecules and atoms. Given that every living creature is assembled from elements forged in the nuclear furnace of some high-mass star from which their progenitor during its final rally before becoming wholly dead Big-Banged its contents into the immense sphere within which lucky Earth—a Goldilocks planet: not too hot, not too cold, just right—would eventually pull itself together from the bountiful debris. Using these raw materials for its countless projects, Earth recycles them through successive generations of rocks, plants, animals, air. And so our planet will continue until our sun, being, alas, too small to go out in explosive style, will in five billion years use its last gumption to bake Earth into pristine sterility, after which Brother Sun will await, together with its by-then-cooled-down-to-freezing planetary acolytes, the collision— already in progress—between the Milky Way and her sister Andromeda, causing our solar monastery to disband forever, albeit a short forever that will lead to a new beginning, a recycling of us and ours in a burst of new stars and maybe another Goldilocks planet or two where once again creatures that breathe may arise to live a final forever, the forever until every star in Mother Universe blinks out, even as its matter, together with the matter of whatever

creatures it had gifted with life, becomes more and more attenuated under Mother's expansion until the dark energy that propels
her runs out and she, every rotund bit, reaches a temperature of
absolute zero, when even her quantum parts will be immobilized
and she, who had been born in a big bang, expires in a whimper.

"Caesar's last breath" is my shorthand for all of these conjunctions, which I have, over my lifetime, secreted in the hallowed space
where I guard my most precious insights. These imbrications,
indeed, stand for the main purpose of my life: being connected, with
honesty and integrity, to the mineral, vegetable, animal, astronomi-
cal, and cosmological worlds, particularly that infinitesimal subset
of the animal kingdom, my fellow humans, with whom I have in
common a wondrously complex brain that gives us access to the
"truth of the Imagination."

Imagine: The calculations that Fermi aficionados make for Caesar's last breath can also be made for every creature that has ever
sojourned on this, our Earth. It means that all my life I have sucked
into my lungs molecules from not only the last breath of animals
and people I have loved, but also from their exhalations at any of
the moments I choose from their biographies: Marissa's and Newton's first yells after gulping air for the first time; Peter's whole-
hearted "Ja" on our wedding day; my mother's pant-pant-blows
as she labored to push me into the world; the wondrous, tiny
spiral galaxy my father created every time he slowly let out the
fragrant smoke from his cigarette; the sorrowful plaints of my
Kalahari grandfather when he came upon his fiancée and her parents dead of the flu during the pandemic of 1918; the awed cries
of my Dutch ancestors when they spotted Table Mountain from
their sailing vessel in the bay; and the joyous vocalizations of my
bi-pedal Paleolithic cousin, Lucy, as she clutched a rock with her
opposable-thumbed fist, smote open a termite mound, and fell

upon the plump and juicy morsels that swarmed from the tunneled habitat.

Imagine: Those who love me breathe me.

Imagine: A final forever. And then: no you, no I, no tomorrow, no yesterday, no names, no memory, no molecules: matter itself released into energy, single photons stretched across light-years of space.

But here and now, still: the magisteria of a mind, the grant of an interval to sound the ordinances of a world without being.

Acknowledgments

I would like to acknowledge Kirstin Scott and Shen Christenson, who not only read and read and read, but also gave me ideas, food, and shoulders to cry on.

I am grateful to my Family Practitioner, Dr. Shana Eborn, who has seen Peter and me through the first five years of my post-diagnosis dementia with patience, empathy, and honest answers. I also would like to acknowledge my neuropsychologist, Dr. Janiece Pompa, who has been utterly generous with timely information and matching support.

I thank my neighbor Diane Bond for generously allowing me to include entries from my Dementia Field Notes about her and her late husband, Bob Bond, and their struggle with his dementia.

I am beholden to my husband, Peter Saunders, for retrieving and editing the photographs and to my daughter-in-law, Cheryl, for creating the illustrations that appear in my book.

I thank Stephen Corey, Jenny Gropp, and Doug Carlson—editors at *The Georgia Review* (GR): Were it not for the extraordinary attention and help they gave my dementia essay during its first launch into print, it may never have progressed along the path toward a book. My gratitude also goes to GR's business manager Brenda Keen, who did the necessary business work for the subsequent reprints.

I am blessed to have Kate Garrick for a literary agent: she knew when to enthuse and when to enjoin me to repair, modify, cut. I am also thankful for Scott Korb and Cathy Jaque's reading of and feedback on the manuscript.

I am thankful for Paul Whitlatch, senior editor at Hachette Books, who believed in my book from the start. Paul led me through the logistics of changing a manuscript into a book with a candor that twins his brilliance. I acknowledge the work of editorial assistant Lauren Hummel, who meticulously attended to even the smallest detail, and the rest of Hachette's A-team who gave their expertise to bring my book into the world.

Notes

v   **Your name is Rock**: The sentence is a praise song chanted to the great Zulu warrior king Shaka, circa 1787 (September 22, 1828). Ezekiel Mphahlele translated it to English. Encyclopaedia Britannica. Copyright 2016, Encyclopaedia Brittanica. Web. Accessed October 31, 2017.

Chapter One: *Telling Who I Am before I Forget*

7   **depriv[ing] sufferers from be[ing] able**: Definition of dementia used by the National Institute of Neurological Disorders and Stroke, National Institutes of Health (NIH). Web. Accessed August 25, 2011.

10   **Call it what you like**: Lewis Carroll, *Alice's Adventures in Wonderland,* 6.57–62. Web. Shmoop University. Accessed August 22, 2014.

10   **When life itself seems lunatic**: *Man of La Mancha,* 1972 musical film based on Miguel Cervantes's seventeenth-century novel *The Ingenious Gentleman Don Quixote of La Mancha.* Directed by Arthur Hiller. Screenplay by Dale Wasserman. Web. IMDb Quotes. Accessed September 8, 2014.

10   **felt the wind on the wing of madness**: "My Heart Laid Bare," *The Columbia Dictionary of Quotations.* Web. *Googlebooks.* August 21, 2014.

Chapter Two: *Quantum Puff Adders and Fractional Memories*

29   Illustration of the limbic system by Cheryl Saunders, as informed by "The Limbic System," Wikipedia.org, and "The Limbic System," from Indiana University's Web Dictionary. Accessed February 10, 2012.

30   **We simply cannot understand thought**: Rebecca Sato, "Vulcans Nixed: You Can't Have Logic without Emotion," Great Discoveries Channel: The Daily Galaxy, May 29, 2009. http://www.dailygalaxy

.com/my_weblog/2009/05/vulcans-nixed-y.html. Accessed December 14, 2011.

30   **to pass on their electrical excitement**: Jonah Lehrer, "The Forgetting Pill," *Wired*, March 2012, 84.

30   **every long-term memory**: Lehrer, as previously cited, 93.

31   **formed and then rebuilt**: This quotation and the ones that follow are from Lehrer, as previously cited, 90.

34   English labels for the various Puff Adder diagrams by Cheryl Saunders.

40   **The faster you go**: "Albert Einstein Quotes," Quoteauthors.com. http://www.quoteauthors.com/albert-einstein-quotes. Accessed September 8, 2014.

40   **Finally, from so little sleeping**: Miguel Cervantes, Chapter 29, "About the Famous Adventure of the Enchanted Boat," *The Ingenious Gentleman Don Quixote of La Mancha*, trans. John Ormsby, 1604. Cervantes Project, Texas A&M University and Universidad de Castilla–La Mancha. Web. Accessed November 6, 2012.

44   **are not of the highly imaginative sort**: John Ormsby, translator's preface: "II. About Cervantes and Don Quixote." *The Ingenious Gentleman Don Quixote of La Mancha*. The Project Gutenberg EBook of Don Quixote, by Miguel de Cervantes. Gutenberg Project. Web. Accessed October 3, 2014.

45   **bounded by the mountains**: Miguel Cervantes, Chapter 14, "Wherein the Dead Shepherd's Verses of Despair Are Set Down, with Other Unexpected Incidents." *The Ingenious Gentleman Don Quixote of La Mancha*, as previously cited.

46   **so I won't die of Truth**: Paraphrase of Ray Bradbury's poem/essay "We Have Our Arts So We Don't Die of Truth," *Zen in the Art of Writing: Essays on Creativity* (New York: HarperCollins, 2015).

Chapter Three: *The Grammar of the Disappearing Self*

50   **because love here has invented language**: Iris Murdoch, *The Black Prince* (New York: Penguin Books, 1973).

51   **prosiness...didacticism, and...reliance on whimsy**: Susan Eilenberg, *London Review of Books* 24, no. 17 (September 5, 2002).

51   **everyone from linguists to neuroscientists to her own husband**: Roger Highfield, "Decline of Iris Murdoch in Her Own Words," *Telegraph*, October 24, 2011.

51   **closer and closer apart**: John Bayley, *Iris: A Memoir of Iris Murdoch* (London: Time Warner Books UK, 2002).

60   **"hugely achieving" woman**: Anne Rowe, "Critical Reception in England of *Iris: A Memoir* by John Bayley," *Iris Murdoch Newsletter* 13 (1999): 9–10.

60   **disclosures about Murdoch**: Pamela Osborn, "'How Can One Describe Real People?': Iris Murdoch's Literary Afterlife," Academia, www .academia.edu/12898733/How_Can_One_Describe_Real_People_Iris _Murdochs_Literary_Afterlife. Accessed September 25, 2016. The point is Osborn's, who cites Derrida in her essay.

60   **Bayley demonstrates**: Anne Rowe, as previously cited.

64   **compartments hermetically sealed**: Mary Gordon, "A True Case of Love That Does Not Alter When It Alteration Finds" [book review], *New York Times*, December 20, 1998.

64   **I always thought it would be vulgar**: John Bayley, *Elegy for Iris* (New York: St. Martin's Press, 1999).

65   **the early stages of Alzheimer's disease on spontaneous writing**: ScienceBlog article from University College London (UCL). "Iris Murdoch's Last Novel Reveals First Signs of Alzheimer's Disease." © 2004. Web. Accessed November 1, 2011.

66   **Susten poujin drom**: Bayley, *Elegy for Iris*, as previously cited.

66   **the grammar of a particular language**: V. S. Ramachandran, *The Tell-Tale Brain: A Neuroscientist's Quest for What Makes Us Human* (New York: W.W. Norton and Company, Inc., 2011).

68   **known to disrupt the brain's**: "Iris Murdoch's Last Novel," as previously cited.

68   **unfamiliar feeling of writer's block**: Ibid.

72   **holiness of the heart's affections**: John Keats, letter to Benjamin Bailey, November 22, 1817. http://www.john-keats.com/briefe/221117.htm.

Chapter Four: *This Is Your Brain on the Fritz*

75   **If your desire is fixed to follow me**: Virgil. Adapted from *Aeneid*, book 2, lines 350–352. Project Gutenberg. http://www.gutenberg.org/ files/228/228-h/228-h.htm. Accessed February 13, 2012.

77   **crinkling it up to fit**: The idea of building the brain out of a modeling substance is from Timothy Verstynen and Bradley Voytek, *Do Zombies*

Dream of Undead Sheep? A Neuroscientific View of the Zombie Brain (Princeton, NJ: Princeton University Press, 2014).

77   **The reptilian brain**: InnerBody.com. Accessed September 9, 2014.

78   **The physical slowing**: Bill Adams, Stray Ideas. http://stray-ideas .blogspot.com. Accessed March 25, 2012.

79   The wrinkled neocortex illustration is by Cheryl Saunders, adapted from the *Journal of Cosmology.* Web. Accessed March 12, 2012.

80   **Comparison of the brain surfaces of various species**: Patricia Kinser, "Brain Structures and Their Functions." *Serendip/Bryn Mawr College.* Web. Accessed January 19, 2012. Illustrations used with the author's permission.

80   **An axon is a long threadlike**: Ka Xiong Charand, "Nerve Cell," HyperPhysics, Georgia State University. http://hyperphysics.phy-astr.gsu.edu/ hbase/biology/nervecell.html. Accessed February 15, 2012.

80   Illustration of the structure of a typical neuron by Cheryl Saunders, adapted from Ka Xiong Charand, as previously cited.

80   **In a living brain, cortical neurons**: Nachum Dafny, "Overview of the Nervous System," Neuroscience Online. http://neuroscience.uth.tmc .edu/s2/chapter01.html. Accessed February 23, 2012.

82   **even as we are elderly and dying**: Eric Jensen, "One of the Five Greatest Discoveries in Neuroscience History Is Being Largely Ignored," Brainbased, Jensen Learning. http://www.jensenlearning.com/news/ discoveries-in-neuroscience/brain-based-teaching. Accessed February 19, 2012.

82   **neurons wither and die**: "Adult Neurogenesis," *Brain Briefings* (Society for Neuroscience), June 2007.

82   **make social judgments**: James Shreeve, "Beyond the Brain," *National Geographic* 207, no. 3 (2005): 22–23.

82   **On a biological level, the acquisition**: Peter S. Eriksson, Ekaterina Perfilieva, et al., "Neurogenesis in the Adult Human Hippocampus," *Nature Medicine* 4 (1998): 1313–1317.

83   **massive state of flux**: Louise Carpenter, "Revealed: The Science behind Teenage Laziness." *Telegraph,* February 14, 2015.

83   **Some scientists have proposed**: "Adult Neurogenesis," *Brain Briefings,* as previously cited.

83   **the idea of brain plasticity**: Michael S. Gazzaniga, *Tales from Both Sides of the Brain* (New York: Ecco, 2015).

88 **wide as a watermelon**: Anne Sexton, "The Big Heart," PoemHunter. http://www.poemhunter.com/poem/the-big-heart-2. Accessed March 27, 2015.

88 **fresh from God**: Charles Dickens, *The Old Curiosity Shop*. Web. Accessed February 26, 2015. The sentence from which I quote reads, "It is not a slight thing when they, who are so fresh from God, love us."

91 **the hole "toward the front"**: Amélie A. Walker, "Neolithic Surgery." *Archeology* 50, no. 5 (1997).

92 **like a bee sting**: "Intracranial Pressure Monitoring," MedlinePlus. https://medlineplus.gov/ency/article/003411.htm. Accessed August 9, 2011.

92 **significant noise and vibrations**: G. Farzanegan et al., "Does Drill-Induced Noise Have an Impact on Sensorineural Hearing during Craniotomy Procedure?" *British Journal of Neurosurgery* 24, no. 1 (2010): 40–45.

93 **Sir Charles Lyell formulated the concept**: Charles Lyell, *The Geological Evidence of the Antiquity of Man* (Philadelphia: George W. Childs, 1863).

93 **there was no unifying theory**: Eric A. Zillmer, Mary V. Spiers, et al. *Principles of Neuropsychology*, 2nd ed. (Belmont, CA: Thomson Wadsworth, 2008).

94 **shellfish brimming with**: Will Block, "Did Shellfish Omega-3s Spur Brain Evolution?" Life Enhancement. http://www.life-enhancement.com/magazine/article/2238-did-shellfish-omega-3s-spur-brain-evolution. Accessed February 12, 2012.

94 **Parke [with] goodly meadows**: Samuel Purchas, *Purchas His Pilgrimage*. Archive.org. https://archive.org/details/purchashispilgri00purc. Accessed October 21, 2014. Coleridge was reading Purchas's book while composing "Kubla Kahn."

95 **The input role of the temporal lobe**: Nachum Dafny. "Overview of the Nervous System," as previously cited.

100 **suffer[ed] a sea-change**: William Shakespeare, *The Tempest*. Ariel's song.

107 **Eternal, and eternal I endure**: Dante Alighieri, *The Divine Comedy: Inferno*, canto 3, lines 8–9, The Harvard Classics (1909–1914), Bartleby.com. http://www.bartleby.com/20/103.html. Accessed March 27, 2015.

111   **Name something else**: Pattiann Rogers, "The Family Is All There Is," EnviroArts. http://arts.envirolink.org/literary_arts/PRogers_Family .html. Accessed February 26, 2015.

118   **the flow of energy between**: Adrienne Rich, *Of Woman Born: Motherhood as Experience and Institution* (London: W. W. Norton, 1976).

119   **danger knows full well**: William Shakespeare, *Julius Caesar*. Cited in Aidan Coleman and Abbie Thomas, *Julius Caesar Googlebooks*. Accessed February 25, 2015.

Chapter Five: *Of Madness and Love I*

123   **he will almost always beat you**: David Owen, "The Psychology of Space," *New Yorker*, January 21, 2013, 29.

123   **local changes in tissue content**: H. J. Rosen, S. C. Allison, et al., "Neuroanatomical Correlates of Behavioural Disorders in Dementia," *Brain* 128, pt. 11 (2005): 2612–2525.

123   **an organ of "mass action"**: Michael S. Gazzaniga, *Who's in Charge? Free Will and the Science of the Brain* (New York: HarperCollins, 2011), 47. Gazzaniga's source is K. S. Lashley, *Brain Mechanisms and Intelligence: A Quantitative Study of Injuries to the Brain* (Chicago: University of Chicago Press, 1929).

130   **This place has only three exits**: René Daumal, *A Night of Serious Drinking*, trans. from the French by David Coward and E. A. Lovatt (Boston: Shambhala, 1979).

130   **As for me and my house**: *As for me and my house*, [we will serve the Lord]. Joshua 24:15, *The Holy Bible*, King James Version (Victoria, Australia: Book Printer, World Bible Publishers, n.d.).

131   **the herd began to follow**: Serge Schmemann. "Russians Tell Saga of Whales Rescued by an Icebreaker," *New York Times*, March 12, 1985.

131   **Turgenev wouldn't do that**: Grace Paley, "A Conversation with My Father," *Enormous Changes at the Last Minute* (New York: Farrar, Straus, Giroux, 1960; 12th printing, 1985), 78.

131   **indescribably offensive**: Brian Foster, "Einstein and His Love of Music," *Physics World*, January 2005.

131   **too personal, almost naked**: "Why Einstein Didn't Like Beethoven (Except the *Missa Solemnis*)," LvB and More, May 4, 2011. http:// lvbandmore.blogspot.com/2011/05/54-why-einstein-didnt-like -beethoven.html. Accessed October 8, 2014.

131   **keep your trap shut**: Brian Foster, as cited above.

131   **the war against Freud's reality principle**: Harold Bloom, "The Knight in the Mirror," *Guardian*, December 13, 2003. https://www.theguardian .com/books/2003/dec/13/classics.miguelcervantes. Accessed November 6, 2014.

132   **our souls touched, quivering**: Adapted from Walt Whitman, "Who Learns My Lesson Complete," *Leaves of Grass* (1855).

144   **It insists on including information**: Gazzaniga, as previously cited, 85.

145   **[e]ach hemisphere was shown four**: Michael Gazzaniga, "The Split Brain Revisited," *Scientific American* 297 (1998): 51–55.

145   **The patient had to choose**: Gazzaniga 1998, as previously cited.

145   **the left hemisphere did not say**: Gazzaniga 1998, as previously cited, 82–83.

147   **Since at the time the term** *quagga*: "The Quagga Revival," The Quagga Project South Africa. http://quaggaproject.org. Accessed October 9, 2014.

155   **an older adult caring for another**: Kyla King, "Report: Alzheimer's Caregivers Suffer Heavy Toll," *Grand Rapids Press*, March 15, 2011.

Chapter Six: *Of Madness and Love II*

158   **had a loving, affectionate relationship**: Pam Belluck, "Sex, Dementia and a Husband on Trial at Age 78," *New York Times*, April 13, 2015. Unless otherwise specified, citations in this entire section of this chapter originate in this article.

159   **Mrs. Rayhons was taken to a hospital**: "Room for Debate: Can People with Dementia Have a Sex Life?" *New York Times*, April 22, 2015.

163   **the intended cure proved**: Gerald Sandler, Delores Mallory, et al., "IgA Anaphylactic Transfusion Reactions," *Transfusion Medicine Reviews* 9, no. 1 (1995): 1.

163   **faking a smile can improve**: Roger Dooley, "Why Faking a Smile Is a Good Thing," *Forbes*, February 26, 2015.

164   **altogether the most free**: Sigmund Freud, "Femininity," *New Introductory Lectures on Psycho-analysis* SE 33. 165. 1933a. *Googlebooks*. Web. Accessed March 28, 2015.

165   **the most comprehensive sex survey**: Marilynn Marchione, "Sex and the Seniors: Survey Shows Many Elderly People Remain Frisky," *New York Times*, August 22, 2007.

165   **Married Couples' Sex Lives Rebound**: Yagana Shah, "Married Cou-
      ples' Sex Lives Rebound—After 50 Years, Study Finds," *Huffington
      Post*, February 19, 2015. http://www.huffingtonpost.com/2015/02/19/
      married-couples-sex-lives-rebound-study_n_6713126.html. Accessed April
      17, 2015.

168   **i carry your heart**: E. E. Cummings, "[I carry your heart with me],"
      Poetry Foundation. https://www.poetryfoundation.org/poetrymagazine/
      poems/detail/49493. Accessed February 11, 2015. This poem originally
      appeared in the June 1952 issue of *Poetry* magazine.

173   **fuller, as if [I] were married**: Nikolai Gogol, "The Overcoat." http://
      intranet.micds.org/upper/ArtDept/Drama/Inspector/Overcoat.pdf.
      Accessed February 27, 2015.

173   **the soul spends**: Luce Irigaray, *The Speculum of the Other Woman* (New
      York: Cornell University Press, 1985).

174   **Donna and I would 'play'**: "Room for Debate," as previously cited.

174   **We just loved to be together**: "Former Iowa Legislator Henry Ray-
      hons, 78, Found Not Guilty of Sexually Abusing Wife with Alzheimer's,"
      Washington Post, April 23, 2015.

175   **didn't South African scientists clone quaggas**: P. Heywood, "The
      Quagga and Science: What Does the Future Hold for This Extinct
      Zebra?" *Perspectives in Biology and Medicine* 56, no. 1 (2013): 53–64.

176   **I understand the world moves**: Banesh Hoffmann and Helen Dukas,
      Albert Einstein, The Human Side: New Glimpses from His Archives (Princ-
      eton, NJ: Princeton University Press, 1979).

178   **injury to a specific part**: Michael Gazzaniga (2011), as previously
      cited.

179   **Many of them remain social**: Benedict Carey, "After Injury, Fighting
      to Regain a Sense of Self," *New York Times*, August 8, 2009.

Chapter Seven: *Makeovers in Extremis*

182   **the deadliest security operation**: Pascal Fletcher, "South Africa's
      'Hill of Horror': Self-Defense or Massacre?" Reuters, August 17, 2012.
      http://www.reuters.com/article/us-safrica-lonmin-shooting-idUSBRE
      87G0MS20120817. Accessed October 15, 2014.

186   **my doctor judged the birth**: *Fairlady*, November 8, 1978, 183–185.

188   **nothing has time to gather**: W. B. Yeats, "Introduction," *Irish Fairy and
      Folk Tales*, ed. W. B. Yeats (New York: Modern Library, 2003).

190   **Living in an increasingly visually mediated**: Shira Tarrant and Mar-
      jorie Jolles, "Introduction: Feminism Confronts Fashion," in *Fashion
      Talks: Undressing the Power of Style* (Albany, NY: SUNY Press, 2012).

197   **each of us engages with fashion**: Beth [no last name given]. "Who Do
      Women Dress For?" Dappered, September 19, 2013. https://dappered
      .com/2013/09/who-do-women-dress-for. Accessed May 23, 2014.

198   **one sequin at a time**: "The Outrageous Lady Gaga," *Glamour* (UK),
      July 7, 2010. http://www.glamourmagazine.co.uk/celebrity/celebrity
      -galleries/2010/07/lady-gaga-interview-quotes/viewgallery/388077.
      Accessed June 21, 2014.

198   **A tomb now suffices**: "Alexander the Great Quotes," Brainy Quote.
      http://www.brainyquote.com/quotes/authors/a/alexander_the_great
      .html. Accessed July 27, 2014. My paraphrase of Alexander the Great's
      supposed epitaph.

198   **Modesty is an attitude**: "Modesty." The Church of Jesus Christ of
      Latter-Day Saints [website]. https://www.lds.org/topics/modesty.
      Accessed July 8, 2014. Immodest note: My son, Newton Saunders, was
      one of the lead developers of the "new" LDS website. Although he was
      one of the top programmers at the company that was contracted to cre-
      ate the website, the LDS committee in charge of the project declined
      his participation because, not being LDS, he didn't have a "Temple Rec-
      ommend," or document that signifies that he has "been found worthy"
      after interviews by church leaders. When the project was subsequently
      plagued with problems and fell behind schedule, Newton's company
      recommended him for the rescue. The church relented. At the project's
      completion, Newton and his wife, Cheryl, an ex-Mormon, were invited
      to dinner with a member of the church's highest governing body, the
      Twelve Apostles, an occasion to which Cheryl wore a dress with a
      décolletage that only met the LDS prescriptions of modesty with the
      aid of a bolero jacket. At the dinner, the Apostle praised Newton not
      only for his excellent work, but also for his thorough knowledge of
      the Mormon scriptures, which had been his task to incorporate in the
      website.

198   **My little lamb, do you know**: As I remember from a phone conversa-
      tion in 1978. Translated from Afrikaans.

209   **Vanity working on a weak head**: Jane Austen, *Emma* (1815). http://
      www.austen.com/emma/vol1ch8.htm. Accessed March 31, 2015.

210   **only mild and lulling airs**: Homer, *Odyssey*, book 4, line 605, The Project Gutenberg EBook of *The Odyssey of Homer*, by Homer, trans. William Cowper. https://www.gutenberg.org/files/24269/24269-h/24269-h.htm. Accessed July 12, 2014.

Chapter Eight: *The Exit That Dare Not Say Its Name*

219   **liked its poetic clumsiness**: Damien Hirst, "The Physical Impossibility of Death in the Mind of Someone Living, 1991," DamienHirst.com. http://www.damienhirst.com/the-physical-impossibility-of. Accessed July 12, 2014. The quote was taken from Gordon Burn and Damien Hirst, *On the Way to Work* (London: Faber and Faber, 2001), 19.

220   **£50,000 for fish**: Carol Vogel, "Swimming with Famous Dead Sharks," *New York Times*, October 1, 2006.

220   **you could tell it wasn't real**: Carol Vogel, as previously cited.

221   **if the glass breaks, we mend it**: Sean O'Hagan, "Damien Hirst: 'I still believe art is more powerful than money,'" *Guardian*, March 10, 2012.

221   **How to Swim with Sharks**: Voltaire Cousteau, "How to Swim with Sharks." Paris, 1812. http://infohost.nmt.edu/~dan/per/quotes/How%20to%20swim%20with%20sharks.htm. Accessed July 7, 2014.

221   **My theory is, be the shark**: Duncan Riley, "Brad Pitt Defends Angelina…and Jennifer Aniston," Inquisitr, January 7, 2009. http://www.inquisitr.com/14595/brad-pitt-defends-angelina-and-jennifer-aniston. Accessed June 28, 2014.

221   **every day you have to deal**: Hans Ulrich Obrist and Damien Hirst, "An Interview," 2007, DamienHirst.com. http://www.damienhirst.com/texts/20071/feb—huo. Accessed July 13, 2014.

222   **Being simultaneously dead and alive**: Adapted from a cartoon from *Omaggio de Venezia*, an art magazine.

222   **The shark is simultaneously life**: Roberta Smith, "Just When You Thought It Was Safe," *New York Times*, October 16, 2007.

222   **he has engaged James Fox**: Catherine Mayer, "Damien Hirst: 'What Have I done? I've Created a Monster,'" *Guardian*, June 30, 2015.

224   **a kernel of identity**: Mitchell Stephens, "To Thine Own Selves Be True: A New Breed of Psychologists Says There's No One Answer to the Question 'Who Am I?'" *Los Angeles Times Magazine*, August 23, 1992.

224   **the self divides the moment**: Mitchell Stephens, as previously cited.

225   **a person could deliberately fashion**: John N. King, *"Renaissance Self-Fashioning: From More to Shakespeare"* [review], *Modern Philology* 80, no. 2 (1982): 183–185.

226   **embedded in the Buddhist teaching**: Robin Cooper (Ratnaprabha), review of David P. Barash's *Buddhist Biology: Ancient Eastern Wisdom Meets Modern Western Science, Western Buddhist Review*, Buddhist Centre, March 7, 2014. https://thebuddhistcentre.com/westernbuddhistreview/ buddhism-biology-interconnectedness. Accessed July 30, 2014.

226   **are one body in Christ**: Romans 12:5.

226   **if each species was created separately**: Ansar Fayyazuddin, "On Darwin's 200th Anniversary," *Against the Current*, no. 143, November– December 2009. http://www.solidarity-us.org/node/2444. Accessed July 20, 2014.

226   **Darwin proposed natural selection**: *Prehistoric Life: A Definitive Visual History of Life on Earth* (New York: Dorling Kindersley Publishing, 2009).

226   **one small step for a man**: Natalie Wolchover, "'One Small Step for Man': Was Neil Armstrong Misquoted?" Space.com, August 27, 2012. http://www.space.com/17307-neil-armstrong-one-small-step-quote .html. Once he had safely returned to terra firma, Neil Armstrong maintained that he had been misheard and that his statement actually contained the article "a" before "man," which is the form in which his declaration makes sense.

227   **people no longer willing to comply**: Johan Malan, "The Dangers of Postmodernism," Bible Guidance, July 2010. http://www.bibleguidance .co.za/Engarticles/Postmodernism.htm. Accessed August 11, 2011.

227   **bereft of origin and purpose**: Robert S. Gall, *"The Self after Postmodernity"* [review], *Journal of the American Academy of Religion* 67, no. 1 (1999): 248–250.

228   **through its discourse, its actions**: Ibid.

228   **most complex and integrated social network**: "Effects of Increasing Digital Connections on Relationships and Community," *The Diane Rehm Show*, August 11, 2014.

229   **in the slow-motion way of Alzheimer's**: "My Father's Brain," *New Yorker*, September 10, 2001.

230   **magnifies the stigmatization already**: Susan M. Behuniak, "The

Living Dead? The Construction of People with Alzheimer's Disease as Zombies," *Ageing & Society* 31, no. 1 (2011): 70–92.

230 **every brain it infects**: Behuniak, as previously cited. 82. She cites Thomas DeBaggio, author of *Losing My Mind: An Intimate Look at Life with Alzheimer's*, and David Shenk, author of *The Forgetting: Alzheimer's: Portrait of an Epidemic*.

232 **significant loss of intellectual abilities**: "Definition of Dementia," MedicineNet.com. http://www.medicinenet.com/script/main/art.asp? articlekey=2940. Accessed July 12, 2014.

233 **characterised by global cognitive impairment**: National Collaborating Centre for Mental Health, "Dementia: The NICE-SCIE Guideline on Supporting People with Dementia and Their Carers in Health and Social Care," 67. https://www.scie.org.uk/publications/misc/dementia/dementia-fullguideline.pdf.

233 **the person is present and approaches AD**: Behuniak, as previously cited, 74. She is citing Thomas Kitwood.

236 **When we were in Chicago in October**: Derek Humphry, *Final Exit: The Practicalities of Self-Deliverance and Assisted Suicide for the Dying* (New York: Delta, 2010).

239 **He was acquitted of assisted**: Derek Humphry and Mary Clement, *Freedom to Die: People, Politics, and the Right-to-Die Movement* (New York: St. Martin's Press, 1998); Euthanasia Research Guidance Organization (ERGO), http://www.assistedsuicide.org. Accessed June 24, 2014.

239 **or even prosecuted at all**: "Kevorkian Released from Prison after 8 Years." NBCnews.com, June 1, 2007. http://www.nbcnews.com/id/18974940/ns/health-health_care/t/kevorkian-released-prison-after-years#.WAfSwZMrKEI. Accessed June 25, 2014.

239 **The last case prosecuted that I could find**: Yasmine Hafiz, "Barbara Mancini Innocent of Assisted Suicide: Nurse Accused of Aiding Father's Death Has Case Thrown Out," *Huffington Post*, February 12, 2014. http://www.huffingtonpost.com/2014/02/12/barbara-mancini-innocent-assisted-suicide_n_4774275.html. Accessed October 13, 2014.

240 **Mature and savvy beyond her years**: Katherine Seligman, "Taking Control: Facing Terminal Diagnosis, Brittany Maynard Plans to End Her Life," *California Magazine*, October 27, 2014. http://alumni.berkeley.edu/california-magazine/just-in/2015-10-05/taking-control

-facing-terminal-diagnosis-brittany-maynard. Accessed March 27, 2014. Seligman quotes Barbara Coombs Lee, president of Compassion and Choices.

240   **the passing of a right-to-die law**: Nicole Weisensee Egan, "Cancer Patient Brittany Maynard: Ending My Life—My Way," *People*, October 27, 2014; Marcia Angell, "The Brittany Maynard Effect: How She Is Changing the Debate on Assisted Dying," *Washington Post*, October 31, 2014; Mollie Reilly, "Right-to-Die Bill Passes in California," *Huffington Post*, September 11, 2015. http://www.huffingtonpost.com/entry/california-right-to-die_us_55f1fbbae4b002d5c078cd6b. Accessed September 24, 2015.

240   **will be seriously considering PAD**: Charles Baron, "Physician Aid in Dying: Whither Legalization after Brittany Maynard?" Health Affairs Blog, March 12, 2015. http://healthaffairs.org/blog/2015/03/12/physician-aid-in-dying-whither-legalization-after-brittany-maynard. Accessed March 26, 2015.

243   **voluntary stopping of eating and drinking**: Nell Lake, "Aid-in-Dying Loophole: Advocates Want You to Know You Can Stop Eating and Drinking," CommonHealth (WBUR), April 18, 2014. http://www.wbur.org/commonhealth/2014/04/18/dying-loophole-stop-eating-and-drinking. Accessed July 15, 2014. WBUR is Boston's NPR station.

244   **After she met any one of these criteria**: Kathleen W. Klein, "On Jackie's Terms: My Mom Was Ready to Die," Hubpages.com, March 20, 2014. Accessed July 17, 2014.

248   **being with family, having the touch of others**: Atul Gawande, "Letting Go," *New Yorker*, August 2, 2010.

251   **the herds of horses**: Gaius Suetonius Tranquillus (ca. 70–ca. 135 CE), *Lives of the Twelve Caesars*, trans. Joseph Gavorse, 80–82. "Suetonius on the Death of Caesar," Livius.org. http://www.livius.org/sources/content/suetonius/suetonius-on-the-death-of-caesar. Accessed August 15, 2014.

251   **I have lived long enough to satisfy**: *The Commentaries of Caesar, to Which Is Prefixed a Discourse Concerning the Roman Art of War*, trans. William Duncan, vol. 2 (1806), 188.

252   **a small parenthesis in eternity**: Thomas Browne, *Christian Morals*,

ed. John Jeffery (London: Henry Washbourne, 1845). Browne's actual phrase reads, "The created world is but a small parenthesis in eternity."

252 **Genesis: In the beginning**: Genesis 1:1–2.

252 **Many African societies**: James Loewen, *Lies My Teacher Told Me: Everything Your American History Textbook Got Wrong* (New York: New Press, 1995), 260.

252 **In the beginning was the word**: Dylan Thomas, "In the Beginning." http://www.poemhunter.com/best-poems/dylan-thomas/in-the-beginning. Accessed August 19, 2014.

253 **The very molecules that make up your body**: Neil deGrasse Tyson, "Beyond the Big Bang," *The Universe* [TV show], September 4, 2007.

253 **man first of all exists**: Jean-Paul Sartre, *Existentialism Is a Humanism* (Cambridge, MA: Yale University Press, 2007).

253 **the future coils**: Marge Piercy, "September Afternoon at Four O'Clock," *The Moon Is Always Female* (New York: Knopf, 1980).

254 **the holiness of [their] hearts' affections**: John Keats, as previously cited.

255 **expires in a whimper**: Neil deGrasse Tyson, "Ends of the World," *Natural History Magazine*, June 1996.

255 **truth of the Imagination**: John Keats, as previously cited.

256 **single photons stretched across light-years of space**: Fraser Cain, "How Will the Universe End?" *Universe Today*, October 17, 2013. http://www.universetoday.com/105588/how-will-the-universe-end. Accessed October 21, 2013.